ADORABLE FAT GIRL GOES ONLINE DATING

BERNICE BLOOM

Bernice Bloom

OOPS, THERE GO MY KNICKERS

Oh, hello. I'm afraid you've caught me at a rather indelicate time; I'm lying on my back, and my silky, cream knickers are discarded somewhere in the room, while a handsome man touches me in the most private of places. Yes, you read that correctly. Me, half naked with a man. He leans closer to me and I wriggle a little, adjusting my hips on the bed.

"Everything OK?" he asks, promising to be as gentle as possible.

"Yes" I say, with a moan in my voice as he hits a particularly delicate part. "Yes, I'm OK."

He looks up and smiles warmly at me, then flicks off his sterile gloves.

"Right, all finished," he says. "That wasn't too bad, was it? Slip your clothes back on and I'll see you in a minute."

God, I hate having smear tests. I mean; I know they're important and lifesaving, and anyone who's had cervical cancer will warn strongly that not having them and getting cancer is a hell of a lot more painful and terrifying than a quick 20 minutes on the doctor's couch every two years...but—bloody hell—I hate them.

I pick up my clothes off the chair, searching through them for my knickers. Where are they? I look back on the chair but there's no sign of them, I turn my trousers inside out, but...no. Christ. Where have they gone? I put the rest of my clothes on, without the knickers, and check one more time before walking out through the curtains, to see the doctor sitting at his desk.

"Before you go, let's just do your blood pressure," he says, inviting me to sit down. He pushes up my sleeve and wraps the cuff around my left arm, inflating the band until it is tight. He peers down at the numbers on the dial and looks at me quizzically. "It's quite high," he says. "Did you know you have high blood pressure?"

"No," I say, and I know what's coming next.

"It might be an idea to try to get your weight down a bit and do a bit more exercise."

"Yes," I reply.

"I know that's boring, but every little pound lost, and every ten minutes of exercise you can do will make a big difference in the end."

"OK. I will try," I say, but it's going to be hard over the next few weeks. I've got Juan Pablo coming to stay. He was one of the dancers I met when I went on a cruise a while ago. We formed the most unlikely friendship after bonding over a 90-year-old called Frank. We ended up stranded in Europe when we missed the cruise back - it was a real fiasco. Anyway, we stayed friends and now he's coming over to visit for the month, and I CAN'T WAIT.

"Are you under any kind of stress?" continues the doctor.

"Anything that's worrying you that could have caused your blood pressure to rise?"

I look at him blankly. Ted and I finished our relationship a few months ago and I'm absolutely devastated. I can't sleep properly, I can't think straight, and I'm self-medicating with Domino's pizzas.

"No," I say. "Everything's just fine."

"You don't look sure," says the kindly doctor, peering over his glasses in a very doctorly way.

"I've had a bit of a tough time, but I've got a good friend coming to stay and will get out of my rut in no time."

"That's good to hear," he says. "I suggest you come back in a couple of weeks just to check your blood pressure is stabilising."

"OK," I say, standing up. "Thanks, doctor. Oh - one thing I should mention. I can't find my knickers anywhere...they must be somewhere in the cubicle."

"Oh, right, fine, of course," he says. "I shall look out for them."

"They are kind of silky…in a cream colour."

"Of course," he says. "If I find them, I'll let you know."

TED AND ME

I walk out onto the street and phone Charlie straight away.

"It was a bloke," I screech at her.

"What?"

"A bloke. Doing my smear test. Why on earth do they have men doing them? It was so bloody awful."

"It might be the only action you're going to get for a while the way you're going, so you better enjoy it."

"Oh, thanks very much," I say. "You're supposed to be my best friend."

"Well, if you won't date anyone, the smear test is going to become a very special time in your life. Was he nice?"

"Not nice like that, no. Nice for a doctor. I can't even remember what he looked like, to be honest. He was kind of nondescript. And I wasn't exactly looking into his eyes."

"No, fair enough. That would be really weird," says Charlie.

"I just don't like it when male doctors do smear tests though. I find it really uncomfortable."

"Me too," said Charlie. "You should have specified that you wanted a woman."

"Yes, but then I just feel like I'm being a huge pain."

"Nah. You should tell them. Definitely tell them next time. Though, like I said, if you're still single next time you have a smear, you might appreciate the attention. You might be asking for a male doctor."

"Will you stop it?" I say. Honestly, she's been moaning at me constantly since Ted and I split up, insisting that I should 'Get Back Out There' and meet someone new before I start seizing up completely. "But I still love Ted," I've said to her, on numerous occasions.

"Well then, go out with him."

"But it wasn't working with him."

"Well go out with someone else, then."

"I don't want to; I love Ted."

"I will come over there and bash you across the head in a minute. You're being very annoying."

The truth is that I do still love Ted, but I don't know whether I want to be with him. Well, when I say that, what I mean is - I want to be with the Ted I first met...Ted who was attentive, funny and a joy to be around. But then our relationship started to feel stale and as if it was continuing out of habit rather than love. Things got more and more difficult.

The thing with Ted was that he worked really hard, which I loved about him, but it meant we hardly ever saw each other, and when we did, he was on his phone half the time. He was always exhausted and didn't want to do anything, and I just got bored by it. I think he did, too...we seemed to get on each other's nerves all the time.

Then, there was the night when it all came to a head. We had spent the evening at his flat bickering and getting annoyed with each other.

It was really dismal and I felt sad, frustrated and angry all at the same time. I remember looking at him and thinking, for the first time in our relationship, I just don't want to be here. I remember looking at my watch and wondering how I could get out of there without it becoming a huge drama.

"You want to go home, don't you?" Ted said.

I looked at him. I didn't want a massive confrontation.

"Be honest with me," he said. "Let's just stop pretending this is working, and be truthful with each other."

I burst into tears at that point, of course, because it was a hideous situation that I didn't want to have to deal with. I loved him. I still love him. There was, and is, no question about that, but I find it frustrating when I am in his company because he doesn't seem to love or cherish me like he used to.

"I do want to go home," I replied, eventually, tears streaming down my face. "But I love you, and want to be with you. I don't want us to split up or anything."

"We don't need to split up," Ted had said. "But I've got quite a lot on at the moment; I need to focus on work. Perhaps a little break would give us both time to think. Let's meet up in a couple of weeks, when I've got through this conference and all the meetings, and we can see how we feel then, OK?"

"OK," I said, reluctantly. "But promise me you won't meet someone else and forget about me forever."

I know, I know. It was deeply pathetic.

"I won't meet anyone else, you idiot. I love you," he replied.

"But perhaps we've been spending too much time together. You keep looking at your watch and clearly really want to be at home, so you should go."

"It's not that I want to be at home," I said, which wasn't strictly true. What was strictly true was that I didn't want him to want me to be at home, and I felt all troubled and upset now he'd suggested it. Is everyone like this, or is it just me?

"Come on, I'll drive you," he insisted.

It felt like all the power in the room had shifted. Now he definitely wanted me to go home, and I really didn't want to. I'd rather sit there feeling miserable, as long as it was in his company, than be at home by myself, feeling alone and unwanted. Tears were pricking at the back of my eyes. I reached for my cardigan and stood up reluctantly, following him to his car like a sulky teenager.

"We're going to be okay, Mary," he said. "Remember that. We're going to be together forever."

"Forever," I'd replied while choking back tears and trying to stop myself feeling anxious and scared. After that, things just seemed to get worse. I went back to my flat and called Charlie, obviously, because a situation like that calls for a chat with your best friend. She came around and stayed with me while we drank wine, ate pizza and I sobbed. "There's nothing to get upset about," she kept saying. "You're still with him, he's just taking some time to get his work projects done, then you'll be back together again - like you should be. Ted'n'Mary."

"Yes," I stuttered, unconvinced, while crying and blowing my nose.

The next two weeks crawled past, then finally, finally, the day arrived. Ted and I were going to meet up and be back on track.

Charlie sent me a cheeky note saying 'I bet he proposes', and my mum phoned to wish me well. It felt like there was quite a lot riding on this date which, with hindsight, wasn't very helpful. I felt under pressure to get the relationship going again as soon as possible.

I got myself all dressed up, of course, and set out to meet him looking as nice as I could.

We met in the pub and when I walked in, he was on the phone and barely acknowledged me. My heart sank. I'd spent an hour and a half curling my hair and £50 on a new dress. He couldn't even say 'hello'.

He seemed so distracted and horrible. I mean, not horrible - because Ted's never horrible- but it felt like he would rather be anywhere else on earth. When I said this to him, he looked angry.

"What do you want me to do?"

"I don't know, be a bit enthusiastic," I said.

He shrugged and told me that he was doing his best, and it was ridiculous that I now wanted to control his mood. He said he'd had a difficult day at work, and I just had to take him or leave him. In that moment I felt like screaming, "leave you then" because I was just so disappointed that he wasn't as excited about seeing me as I was him.

I'd been looking forward to this moment every day for the past fortnight and now he was ruining it.

We sat there in silence after that; Ted sipping his pint and me getting crosser and angrier, and more and more upset.

Then he looked at his watch. "Come on, let's go," he said.

He dropped me home, gave me a peck on the cheek, and said he had to get back and have an early night because he had to go to work the next day.

I felt like I'd been shot. I'm sure my heart dropped a little. I know this is pathetic and I know it doesn't necessarily mean you are being rejected when a guy says he's got a lot of work on. But it hurt. Ted never had too much work on to stay the night when we first met; now he did. Given we hadn't seen each other for two weeks and we were fighting to keep the relationship going, he could have stayed.

I had pictured him turning up with a big bouquet of flowers, whisking me off somewhere wonderful and having a picnic that he'd prepared. Instead he'd asked me to meet him in the local pub, spent half the time on the phone then dropped me off without wanting to come in. Now, come on - I know I can be a drama queen at times, but that's not right, is it? That's not how someone behaves when they're in love with you.

He'd made me feel as if he was only there because he had to be, and not because he was desperate to see me.

After the paltry kiss on the cheek he left and I went and lay on my bed. Later I sent him a text saying I realised he was very busy at work, and maybe we should leave it for now, and aim to meet up in a few weeks' time. Then I ignored his texts for a while, didn't take his calls, and by the time we spoke to each other, a month later, I said that I didn't feel the same about him. That was about a month ago. Now we're in limbo; we've sort of split, but nothing's been clarified.

I remember one time, near the beginning of our relationship, when we had a row and he turned up at my flat and sprinkled rose petals everywhere. Not this time; he just stayed away.

My friends have been disappointed in him, which is why they're urging me to get out there and meet someone new. But...I don't know.

I kind of just want to be with Ted.

THE ARRIVAL OF JUAN

It's 6pm and Charlie and I are at Heathrow airport awaiting the arrival of the lovely Juan Pedro. I can't believe he's coming to stay; it's been so long since I last saw him, though we have been Skype-ing regularly and we've kept up with each other's news.

I've been trying to explain to Charlie what Juan is like...how he's very flamboyant and peacock-like but also warm, tender and very kind. I've explained that he's great fun and a bit crazy, but also the sort of person you can rely on. She's heard me talk about him in the past, of course. When I came back from my three-week cruise, I couldn't stop talking about him, and showed her all the incredible pictures of him; dancing on the stage in his sparkly trousers, and out on the town at night in his sparkly trousers.

"He looks just as glamorous off stage as he does on," said Charlie.

"Yep...just you wait," I replied.

The truth is that Juan is an absolute nutter. He is the loveliest, kindest man – flamboyant, loud and gorgeous – but also a complete nutter. In short, he is exactly what a girl needs when she's been suffering from heartbreak. I'm dying to introduce him to Charlie.

It has already flashed up on the board that his flight has landed, so now we're just waiting for the sight of my glamorous Spanish friend amidst the sea of returning holidaymakers in their ill-fitting shorts and raspberry-ripple legs. Then, he's there – as magnificent as I remember him. He's got white blond streaks through his dark hair which puts me in mind of a badger, but besides that he's exactly the same. He wears mirrored sunglasses, and wiggles along in trousers that are a couple of sizes too small for him. It means that every step he takes is tiny, so he's doing lots of them to keep up with everyone, dragging his bag on wheels behind him, causing all eyes to swivel in his direction, just the way he likes it.

He's wearing tight black and red striped trousers which finish just above his ankle, with red loafers, a red belt, and a skin-tight white T-shirt. In his left hand he clutches a bright red, felt Fedora, and in his right hand is his immaculate, bright red case. He must be the only man in the world whose suitcase matches his hat. You've got to give the man credit; he does nothing by halves on the sartorial front.

"Hello, my gorgeous angel," he says, thrusting his bag at Charlie, and wrapping his arms around me. He seems so genuinely pleased to see me that it really cheers me up.

"I have been looking forward to this day for so long," he says. "You look magnificent as ever. How have you been, my little chickadee?"

I don't answer his question because I don't want to ruin the moment with talk of my collapsed relationship. Instead I turn to Charlie and introduce him. She smiles warmly at him as she takes in the splendid sight before her.

Juan hands me his hand luggage before looking Charlie up-and-down. He studies her from the front, the sides and the back, and tells her she is very beautiful and that if he weren't gay, he would marry her straight away. She looks delighted and tells him that were he not gay, she would be thrilled to accept his proposal.

"We are the three amigos," he says, striding off across the concourse. Charlie is pulling his case and I am holding his hand luggage as we sprint after him. Juan, meanwhile, throws his bright red hat onto his head at a rakish angle, and steps out ahead of us. If only he had a cane, he'd be like Willie Wonka leading us through the chocolate factory.

It's about a half hour drive back from Heathrow to my flat, but Juan manages to embarrass us about fifty times during the course of it, leaning out of the window and doffing his hat at everyone we pass. He is shouting at people and telling them that he likes their coat, hair or car. We finally pull into my road and I'm giddy with relief.

"Well, that was pleasant," he says. "I met lots of new people. Which apartment is yours?"

"It's this one," I say, pointing to the rather rickety white gate leading to steps down to my neighbour's flat, and a couple of steps up to mine. "Mine's the top flat."

"Flat," says Juan to himself. "Top flat. We're definitely in England now, aren't we?"

It's left to Charlie and I to unload his bags from the car and take them inside, while Juan surveys the street and seems quietly to approve of it.

"Nicer than I thought," he says, hugging me affectionately.

"What do you mean, 'nicer than you thought'? Did you imagine me living in a dump?"

"No, I knew you'd live somewhere lovely, but I hadn't imagined it being so very English and so very quaint."

"Ahhh," I say, hugging him back. I'm inordinately fond of my little flat, and I'm glad he likes it too.

Once we're inside, I head for the kitchen and pull a bottle of wine out of the fridge, pouring generous amounts into each of the glasses. I can hear Charlie and Juan chatting away in the sitting room and it gives me great joy that they are enjoying each other's company so much. It's always great, isn't it...when you know people from different areas of your life, then when they meet, they really get on.

It's such a joy.

I walk out with the drinks, and Juan demands that he see the bottle before he will lift the glass to his lips.

"You haven't got a clue what one wine is like over another," I say.

"No, but I have to keep up the pretence," he says, mimicking a British accent. Having feigned a check of the label, he takes a huge gulp of his wine and sits back.

"How's the love life, then? Back with Ted yet?" he asks.

"Nope. It's over," I say. "I haven't seen him for months and he's not remotely interested in me."

"But are you interested in him?" Juan asks.

"No," I lie, avoiding Charlie's eye.

"Is there someone new in your life?"

"No. There's no way anyone would be interested in me. Look at me," I say.

"What? You're beautiful. Any man would be proud and honoured to be with you."

"Well, no one has made any approaches to me. I'm going to be old and grey and living here surrounded by cats in twenty years."

"You will be if you carry on sulking like this," says Charlie. She turns to Juan. "I can't get her to come out, she should be meeting new men and having fun, not hanging about at home hoping that he comes back to her."

"I've not been hanging around at home," I say. "I've been chilling."

"I think we need to get her back out into the world of men, Juan," says Charlie. "In fact, what we need is for Mary to get herself internet dating - meeting new people and having fun."

"Well, of course. Por supuesto," says Juan. "Let's get her online immediatamente."

By the time the second bottle has been consumed, a plan has been hatched. It's a plan that has been cooked up by Charlie and Juan for their amusement although they are trying to convince me that this is all for me...to give me a bright and interesting couple of weeks.

"So, just to confirm," slurs Charlie. "Juan and I will put together a profile of you, then put it onto dating websites and come up with dates for you over the next two weeks."

"Right," I say. "Do I get to see the profile you put together?"

There's a small whispered discussion and the verdict comes back. Yes, I can see my profile, but the choice of men is entirely theirs, and I will only be given a small picture and a few details about each one before meeting them for a date.

"What's your lucky number?" Juan asks.

"I don't know…three."

"Oh, that's no good. Any other numbers?"

"Why do you want to know?"

"I just do. OK, look - we'll multiply three by three to get nine."

"Right," I say. I don't know what's happening now.

"Nine will be your lucky number. We will organise nine dates for you over the next two weeks. All you have to do is turn up. OK?"

"Oh God. OK," I say, mainly because it might be fun, and it would be nice to go on some dates, but also because I've drunk way too much wine and saying 'yes' is easier than fighting my way to a 'no'.

"I'm going to bed," I say, staggering to my feet. "See you in the morning."

"Yep," says Juan, pouring the remainder of the wine into his glass and Charlie's glass. "We've got a bit of talking to do, but we'll see you tomorrow."

I give them both a big hug good night, and tell Juan how pleased I am that he's here, then I waddle into my room and collapse on the bed. Oh Lord. What on earth have I just agreed to?

PLANNING

I am up first the next morning and head into the kitchen to get a coffee. Juan is fast asleep on the sofa rather than in the spare room. I peer into the room he should be in - my tiny box room - and there's Charlie, fast asleep on the bed. How chivalrous of him. I don't know what time they were up until last night, but they both look exhausted.

I go over to the computer and hit the return key. There in front of me, in all its glory, is the profile they created last night. There's a rather rough-looking photograph, but they have written nice things about me. I'm pleased to say that they have put the profile together as themselves, saying that they are great friends of mine and think I'm the loveliest person ever. They say I'm kind and funny and want to be loved. That makes me feel all teary. I suppose I do want to be loved. I guess everyone does. Certainly everyone embarking on internet dating. Why the hell would you put yourself through all this if you weren't hoping to find love at the end of it?

The profile continues by saying that I'm a family person and a loyal friend and I'm a one-man woman. That really stops me in my tracks because it makes me think straight away of Ted: lovely, kind and smiley Ted.

Lower down there are descriptions of the sort of man they think I'd like to meet: big, strong, kind and loving. All true, but - again - it feels like they are describing Ted.

"Oy, what are you doing?" says Charlie, appearing in the room in my nightshirt which is about four times too big for her, making her look all little girl lost and pretty despite the fact that she's still wearing yesterday's makeup and her hair is all crazy and matted.

"Nothing," I say, jumping back from the screen as if she's caught me selling babies on the dark web. "Nothing at all."

"Dios mio," shrieks Juan, arising from his slumber to find me at the computer. "You must not see the men."

"Calm down - I just looked at the profile which you said I could look at anyway. I didn't look at any men. The profile's nice, by the way."

"Thanks," said Charlie. "Though we were blind drunk when we did it, so we should check it makes sense."

"Shall I make some breakfast?" says Juan, sitting up sharply before lying back down again and holding his head.

"I'll do it," says Charlie, seeing him in distress.

"Have you moved in or something?" I say to her.

"Well, it's fun here," she replies. "I'll go if you want me to."

"I'm only joking," I say. "You can stay as long as you like."

"Good, cos I like plotting with Juan. I want us to find you someone lovely. Someone who makes you smile."

"Hmph," I reply. "Anyway, I thought we could go out for breakfast. I have to pop into the centre to collect some tax form. PD11 or something. I can't do my tax return without it. I thought we could pop in and collect that and have breakfast at the centre...there's a really nice cafe and I get 50% off."

"Sure," say Charlie and Juan. But no one moves. Charlie is sitting on the end of the sofa and has her legs under Juan's duvet. There's no sign of any of us going anywhere for a while, so I join them too, and the three of us just sit there, all warm and cosy in my little flat with a big duvet over us, enjoying life. Enjoying each other and the power of friendship. I think we could have stayed there all day were it not for my stomach rumbling loudly, followed by Charlie's rumbling too, then Juan declaring that he hadn't eaten anything the day before – his entire calorie consumption had come from the gallon of wine he drank last night.

"Come on then, to the garden centre," I say. And we all rush off to get changed. Now, I'm very proud of my friends, I really am, and I'm delighted to introduce them to my work mates. But when Juan emerges in a blue silk shirt, open to the waist and skin tight trousers with bright blue peacock feathers all over them, with white, sparkly loafers, I do wonder what on earth my colleagues will say. Juan is such an incredibly exotic creature...it's like he's been beamed down from another planet. The people at work are – how do you say this? – very much of this planet. They are not very exotic at all.

In the end, of course, he is the biggest hit imaginable with everyone, and has them all in stitches as he tells them about how we met on the cruise.

"And now I am going to help her find the man of her dreams," he says.

"Ohhhhh..." they all reply. "How are you going to do that?"

"Internet dating," he says proudly.

"Oh, you have to be careful of that," says George, the young lad who works in houseplants, but is desperate to move over to hardware, so can usually be found amongst the hammers and screwdrivers, leaving the spider plants entirely to their own fate.

"Why?" I ask.

"My mate went on some online dates. He met a girl for dinner and they had a lovely time, until the end of the meal," replies George.

"There was food left over so the waiter asked whether they would like to take it with them. My mate says: 'No thank you,' because - like - they are on a date. But the girl says 'yes' straight away, and adds: 'My boyfriend can have that. I won't have to cook for him tonight'."

"No!" We all squeal in harmony.

"Yes," replies George confidently. "And it wasn't the only thing...The next day he woke up and went to his car and the windscreen was smashed and two of his tyres were flat. There was a message saying "don't mess with my girlfriend". He'd never do internet dating again after that."

"Not as bad as what happened to my mate's dad," says Trevor, coming out of the storeroom and joining us for a chat. He stinks of cigarettes, and I feel like telling him that if he gets caught smoking in the storeroom Keith will sack him. But I am more eager to hear his internet dating story than I am to save his career, so I let him get on with his tale.

"My mate's mum died of cancer, and a few years afterwards his dad decided he wanted to meet someone new, so he went onto the internet and made a date with this lady. He was so nervous before the date, he almost cancelled it, but my mate assured him that it was a good way for older people to meet new partners, so he went ahead.

"They met for a drink at a pub, and got on really well. My mate's dad thought she was a cracking bird, so he asked her if she fancied going for dinner. He pulled out all the stops and took her to that nice hotel, you know the one on the river? Well, anyway, they went in there and he pulled out her seat for her and everything - being all gentlemanly, he was. She sat down and he went and sat down opposite her, then she had a kind of coughing and choking fit. She couldn't stop coughing. He kept asking if she was OK, but then she suddenly fell face down onto her plate.

"He wasn't sure whether she was doing some sort of comedy turn to start with, but then he realised she wasn't moving. He wasn't quite sure what to do. He went around the table to see whether she was all right, and a waiter came over to help, but when they tried to lift her face, it was no good at all. Anyway, to cut a long story short – she was dead."

"Dead? What the hell sort of story is that? What do you mean she was dead?" I ask.

"Brown bread. I swear on my life it's true, he couldn't believe it...

"The woman was dead on the spot. They called an ambulance and everything, and he went with her to the hospital, but she was dead before the ambulance even got there. It's a shame really, because he got on really well with her sons when they turned up. He said they were a really nice family. I think he went to the funeral and everything, and fitted in well with them, so it's a shame she died."

SHOPPING

"Well, that was sobering," I say to Charlie and Juan as we sit in the café with our large breakfasts in front of us. "What if someone dies on me?"

"Not going to happen," says Juan. "We will select only young, fit, healthy specimens...not people who will die."

"If they are young and fit, they won't fancy me: look at me," I say.

Juan looks at me and shrugs. "You are gorgeous...any man can see that. I'm not sure about the outfit you're wearing. It looks like you are in your pyjamas, but besides that - you are lovely."

"I always wear T-shirts and leggings when I'm not out in the evening," I respond. "They are comfy."

"I know you always wear T-shirts and leggings. I looked through your wardrobe earlier...God help me - where do you keep your real clothes?"

"I like dressing like this. These clothes are comfy."

"Yes, they may be comfy, but are they alluring...will they catch the man of your dreams?"

"No, I guess not," I say. "But if the man of my dreams doesn't like me like this, the relationship will never work, because this is how I dress. He has to like me for me."

"I understand that," says Juan. "But you have to make an effort. The man who comes to meet you might like to hang around at home naked, with his hairy balls hanging out; it doesn't mean he should come on a date like that, does it?"

"Christ, no," I reply.

"Well then...you need to make an effort just as he needs to make an effort."

"I guess…" I say, trailing off, because I know he's right, but the thought of a man turning up for a date with his balls hanging out has made me feel a little queasy. I take a large sip of tea.

Juan starts calling up various outfits on his phone that he thinks I will like, while I run my thickly buttered toast through the bean juice on my plate. God, I love breakfasts. I'm just filling my mouth with the joyful combination of beans, butter and toast when my phone rings and Dave's delicious face pops onto the screen. Dave is my neighbour; he lives in the flat below me and is staggeringly good looking...like a young Elvis Presley meets a young Jose Mourinho. I went through a phase of being quite obsessed with him and going down to his flat every now and again and letting him do naughty things to me even though he had a girlfriend and would throw me out as soon as she called. But now we've settled into a warm friendship and I enjoy his company. He'd a decent guy beneath the chiseled jaw, green eyes and ridiculously long eyelashes.

"What the hell was going on last night?" he says. "Was there a party that you didn't invite me to?"

"No, just a couple of friends were over - you know Charlie, and my friend Juan from Spain."

"Oooo, is she pretty? I like Spanish girls. Tell her to come down with her castanets tonight."

"Juan is a man," I say, and there's a moment of silence while Dave recalibrates as the thought of a night with a lovely Spanish girl disappears from his mind.

"What are you doing?" he asks. "Are you at work today?"

"No, I'm having breakfast with the guys, then I think we're going shopping in Kingston."

"We are definitely going shopping in Kingston," shouts Juan.

"Can I join you in my lunch hour?" says Dave. I don't think he has any desire to come shopping with me, but he's clearly curious about my friends.

"You don't want to come shopping with us," I say. "Honestly, we're just going to get a few outfits because I'm going to start internet dating."

There's a silence on the end of the phone.

"Dave? Are you still there?"

"Internet dating?"

"Yep, Charlie and Juan are finding men for me and I'm going to go on a series of dates. They think it's important that I get back out there after Ted."

Charlie and Juan are nodding at me as I speak.

"So, it's completely over with Ted?" asks Dave. "I thought you two were bound to get back together."

"Well, yeah, for now it is," I say. "I don't know - I guess relationships are tough, aren't they?"

"Hell yes," says Dave. "I avoid them like the plague. Internet dating is no push over though...you meet some right characters on there. Make sure you don't let anyone get too close until you know them."

"Right," I say. I don't know what else to reply. I mean - how could I let them get close before knowing them?

"People pretend to be something they're not. There's a lot of catfishing on there."

"Catfishing?"

"Yes. Or certainly kitten-fishing."

"Oh my God, Dave. What the hell are you talking about? I've never heard of any of these things."

"Do you want me to come up tonight and tell you all about it?"

"Yes please," I say. "Come up when you get back from work and you can meet Juan."

"OK, see you around 6pm," he says. "Happy shopping."

Charlie has to leave for work, so Juan has me all to himself for our shopping trip. He moves us from the table to the wicker chairs by the window and sits back, wrapping his legs around each other in a most unnatural fashion. He's kind of double-folded them so his legs look like they're plaited together.

"Is that comfortable?" I ask him. "You know - with your legs all tied in knots."

"Perfectly," he says, unravelling them elegantly. "Now - stop changing the subject and stop trying to distract me. We need to get some sexy outfits to throw into that wardrobe along with the oversized sweatshirts, baggy trousers and loose-fitting dresses."

"I did have some nice clothes. When I first met Ted, I

dressed up all the time, but then I just got lazy, and it's hard when you're fat, Juan. You'll see when we go to the shops. There's hardly anything to buy and my first thought when buying something new is not, 'will it flatter my body' but, 'will it hide my body?'. If it won't I don't buy it, it's as simple as that."

I always buy clothes that are much larger than I am because I don't want them to even skim my bulges, I want them to hang over the top, not touching any lumps or bumps.

My clothes disguise my non-attributes rather than drawing any attention to my attributes. I try to explain this to Juan, and he brings his legs back over one another until they are all knotted up again, shaking his head as he does so.

"You're going to be online dating; you're going to be meeting new men who need to see how gorgeous you are. They don't want to see a woman's head on top of a tent."

"OK," I say.

"So, it's time to go shopping?"

"Yes," I reply.

A short bus ride later, and we are speed walking through Kingston, Juan Pedro is striding ahead. I notice that his shoes clickety-clack like a tap dancer as he walks. I shuffle along behind in my large T-shirt and baggy tracksuit bottoms. I did my hair and makeup this morning before leaving for breakfast, but I haven't shaved my legs for God knows how long, and I'm not looking forward to parading around a shop with my fat arse and hairy legs for all to see.

As we pass Marks & Spencer, I run to catch Juan. "There are clothes in here that I can fit into," I say.

He looks disdainfully at the shop window then at me. "We can do better," he says.

"But the shop has my sizes in. You're being really kind,

taking me shopping, but most of the shops don't have clothes to fit me."

"What about this one?" says Juan, storming into a little independent store, full of frilly, lacy pieces of clothing that would struggle to wrap themselves around someone half my size. I'm not sure I'd get the waist of some of these dresses around my wrist.

"Darling," he says, storming up to the assistant, and complimenting her on her jewellery. "Wonderful, magnificent," he is saying." Now, I want you to dress my beautiful friend here in the most gorgeous clothing you have...clothing that will make her look like a desirable siren."

"OK," says the woman, looking bewildered at the forceful nature of Juan, and slightly dubious about the task ahead of her.

"Can I check what size you are?" she says, moving towards the rails, and flicking through the clothing, whilst she must know, beyond any doubt, that she has nothing there that will go anywhere near to fitting me.

"I'm about an 18 to 20," I say. "Do you have clothes that big?"

"Of course they do," says Juan. "It would be madness if they didn't. They have to be able to dress people, don't they?" He looks expectantly at the woman who has not looked up from where she is frantically searching through the rails.

"You could try this 12?" she says. "These are quite generous."

Quite generous? I look at the flimsy item in her hand and at Juan.

"Try it on," he urges.

"Juan, it's at least four sizes too small."

He sighs deeply and looks at the shop assistant. "Why are you giving us clothes that don't fit her?" he asks.

"We don't have any clothes in your friend's size," she says.

"Why? Do you think my friend is fat?" he asks.

My cheeks flush with heat.

"No," says the assistant, now squirming with embarrassment. "No, no, not at all."

"Then why do none of your clothes fit her? Is this a children's shop?"

"No sir," replies the assistant.

"Then it is simply a bad shop, no?"

"Well, it just caters for the slimmer lady."

"It caters for people who don't eat?"

"Yes," says the assistant. I have to say; I'm feeling quite sorry for her by now.

"Then, you should be based in Africa, yes? You should be somewhere where there are people who have little to eat. They would welcome your services, no? Let's move this shop to somewhere where they need tiny clothes because they have no food, they have to walk ten miles every day for water and they are living in poverty."

The assistant just looks at him blankly.

"Or you would like to stay here?" he offers.

She nods.

"You want to stay here, in this country?"

"Yes," she says.

"Then make clothing for the people who live here in this country. Make clothes for actual real people...people who have money to eat and who enjoy to dine out with friends, people who have lives and families, and babies. People who have real lives."

"OK," she says.

"Good," says Juan, spinning and heading out of the shop. He

pauses by the rack of size zero dresses and turns back for one final assault.

"This is absurd," he says, holding the item into the air. "Any woman who starves herself to fit into this needs to have her head examined. These clothes are for ugly people, soulless, sad and desperate people whose hopes and dreams can be bottled and bagged and hung in their wardrobes. Tragic."

Then, we're off, stomping out of there while a red-faced assistant watches us go.

"You're the best," I say to him, when we're out on the street. "Just - the best."

"I know," he says, giving me a hug. "Shall we go back to that Mark and Spencer place, or whatever it was called?"

"Yep," I reply.

I swear to God; every woman needs a Juan.

DIRE WARNINGS FROM DOWNSTAIRS DAVE

Dave arrives bang on the dot of 6pm, clutching a clipboard like he's come to do a mortgage evaluation of the property, or measure up for double-glazing, or something.

"Evening," he says, striding into the sitting room to greet Charlie and Juan.

"Good God alive," says Juan, practically swooning. "Who in the name of all the angels in heaven are you?"

"I'm Dave. I live downstairs," he says.

"Why, you're beautiful."

"Err...thank you," he says. He's gone a very bright red and looks nervous.

"And, look at you being all professional with your clipboard and smart trousers."

"I've come from work," he says, defensively. "Unlike you, I can't go to work in peacock feather trousers and a silk blouse."

"Then you're in the wrong job," says Juan, "because you

would look completely spectacular in these trousers…preferably with me still in them."

Dave gives Juan a look which forces him to recoil and move to the far side of the room, while I hand Dave a beer and tell him to ignore Juan. It's quite a strange moment - protecting Dave from the predatory Juan, when Dave is the ultimate predator.

I explain that Charlie and Juan have arranged a pile of dates and I am going to go on them without really knowing who I'm going to meet.

"I guess it will be fun," I say, without much conviction.

"Do you have lots of nice things to wear?"

"Yes," I reply. "I've got a great cream shift dress, lovely high-heeled black boots, black trousers that don't make me look like a horse and a frilly blouse. Oh, and also – a lovely, elegant cream jumper and lots of pearl necklaces that make me look like Madonna circa 1986. It should be good fun. I'm quite into the idea of internet dating now."

"You've just got to make sure you're safe – that's the most important thing," he says.

"Yes – so tell me about all the dangers lurking out there."

"It's not so much that it's all desperately dangerous or anything, it's just that it's a very different way of dating, and people can act differently. You need to be aware of what could happen."

"OK, fire away then."

"Let's start with 'stashing'," he says, warming to his theme. "Ever heard of that?"

None of us have.

"OK, well this is very common in internet dating...it's when you've been seeing someone but they are also seeing other people so they try to keep you at arm's length…they never make you 'official'. This allows them to keep their options open, and date other people if they want to. If you meet someone like this, who does this to you - you must do the same - date lots of different people, and not just the one guy. OK?"

"OK," I say. "But - I'm not wild about dating one new person, let alone a whole load."

"Treat them the way they treat you, honey," says Charlie.

"OK," I say, sounding and feeling very unsure.

"What's troubling you?" asks Juan. "You've gone all quiet."

"Just the whole dating thing," I say. "It's so hard. How do you know what a guy's doing?"

"You have me here to explain," says Dave.

"No, I mean - what if a guy's being cautious and taking it slowly because he likes me, and doesn't want to move too fast? I could easily mistake his intentions and think I'm being stashed."

"No - honey, you'll know. You'll feel it. You have to go with your gut instincts on these things. I'd say that's where people go wrong with internet dating. They trust the person on the other side of the computer and not their own instincts. I think it's because it's much harder to tell when someone's lying if your main correspondence with them comes through non-verbal communication.

"If you're going to go down this path, you have to listen to your gut."

"OK," I say. "So, if I think he might be behaving oddly, I have to ask myself why."

"Yes - exactly. And it may be that he's taking his time to introduce you to people…your gut will tell you."

"Right, OK, what other things are there?"

"Ghosting, obviously…"

"I've heard of ghosting, but not really sure what it is..."

"It's one of the most well-known dating terms out there. It just means that someone you've been seeing, or talking to for a while, suddenly disappears and stops contacting you."

"It happens all the time in the gay community," says Juan. "All the time. Drives me nuts. Smile, shag, ghost. Start again. No relationships."

"Yeah, it's horrible," says Charlie. "Instead of having a break-up conversation with you, the guy you're seeing just vanishes without trace. You could have been dating someone a few days, or a few months, but one day they simply disappear. They don't return your texts, and may even block you. It's cowardly."

"Then one day they might suddenly come back," says Juan. "They've been off and dated some other poor sod, then realise they like you after all, so they pop up on your phone months later. It's called zombie-ing when someone who dismissed you rises from the dead and comes back at you. They often act like nothing happened. An innocuous "hey" might appear on WhatsApp, or something similar to tempt you to reply.

"Thanks to social media, the zombie might also try to get back into your life by following you and liking your posts on Instagram and Twitter. Even if you like the guy and want to get back with him, you have to say 'no' to zombies or they will just do it again."

"OK, so that's ghosts and zombies, are there any others? And do you want another beer?"

"Loads," replies Dave.

"Loads more dating advice or loads more beer?"

"Both," he says, before launching into an explanation of 'benched'.

"OK, so this is a bit like the sports team where you're not

first choice but are left on the bench as a reserve. You find yourself being someone's back-up option as they continue to look around for their ideal woman. They may come back to you if nobody better comes along, but that doesn't give one high hopes for the relationship, does it?"

"No," I say. I've got myself a pen and paper now because I feel I ought to be writing all this down.

"There's catch and release as well," says Dave. "This is what people who love the thrill of the chase do. They'll put all their effort into flirtatious texts, and trying to date you, until they "catch" you. But once they've caught you, they lose interest and go looking for someone else to chase.

"Then I should also mention bread crumbing - when somebody seems to be pursuing you, but really, they have no intention of being tied down to a relationship. They send you nice texts and friendly messages, like bread crumbs, to keep you interested in them, but they're not really interested in you. Next there's catfishing – I mentioned this one before – it's when someone lies about who they are, so they could use a completely wrong photo, give you the wrong job or age or height. It's when people lie about who they are...because they can: because this is the internet."

"And what about kitten fishing? Is that the same sort of thing?"

"Yes – it's when a guy presents himself in an unrealistically positive way. A photo that's out of date or edited, or lying about his age. Not all-out lying, like cat fishing, but definitely giving a false impression."

"I see. But aren't you just going to find out that they are lying as soon as you meet them?"

"Yep, which is why you find that some of these guys won't want to meet you."

"Gosh – this sounds terrifying."

"It can be. When you take into account slow fade, cuffing season and pulling pig…"

"I think that's enough, to be honest," says Juan, interrupting. "I don't think we need to completely put her off."

"OK, but she was interested."

"Yeah, and that's enough."

"OK," I say, and I think I agree with Juan – that's probably enough.

FIRST DATE: DARREN

Here we go then, date number one and I couldn't be happier. Actually, that's a lie, I could be much happier if I was left alone and could sit in front of the telly drinking wine and eating pizza while feeling miserable about Ted. But I can't do that, so instead, I'm off out on a date.

"Bye, have a lovely time," shout Charlie and Juan through the living room window as I walk down the steps and out through the gate.

"Bye," says Dave, coming out of his flat and waving at me. I feel like I'm in Balamory or something. "Remember everything I've taught you," he adds.

"Sure," I say, speeding up as I walk down the road towards the bus stop.

I feel a bit trussed up, to be honest. I'm in higher shoes than I'd normally wear, and the new cream dress with the pile of pearl necklaces. I can see, objectively, when I look in the mirror, that it's a good look and if anyone else was wearing it I'd think they looked very nice.

But the necklaces are not me. Not at all.

When the bus comes, I climb aboard, take a seat and hastily take off the necklaces, shoving them into my handbag. I feel better already.

I pull out the piece of paper, on which the details of the man I'm going to see, have been scrawled. He's single, having been married in the past, works for the Postal Service, which I guess means he's a postman. That's all right. That's a proper, solid, down to earth sort of job, isn't it? Someone you can rely on. It's job I understand, not like all these people who say they work in "data marketing" and "digital development". What is that? What an earth does all that mean?

"I'm vice president of crockery cleanliness."

No, mate, you wash the dishes.

Anyway, the point is that Darren is straightforward. He's a postman and he is looking to find someone to fall in love with. Yay.

In his picture he doesn't look like the most handsome man who ever walked the Earth, but then I'm no Beyoncé either, so that's fine.

He looks friendly and approachable and as if he'd be good fun and reliable. What more could a woman ask for?

As the bus trundles along, I fantasise to myself that this could be the one. He might be the man I've been waiting all my life to meet.

Then I can cancel all those other online dates, and just get to know him. He can come around to my house once he's finished his postal round and we can eat pizza (most of my fantasies involve pizza). It will be perfect.

We are meeting at the Coach and Horses, the lovely pub on the green in Esher, so it's not too far for me to go, and easy enough for me to get back from if he turns out not to be my Prince Charming after all. I pull out my compact, and touch up my makeup, fiddling with my hair to see whether I can make it look any better without making it look too 'fussed with'.

Then we are here. I step cautiously off the bus in my high heels, and I clip clop towards the pub. I feel nice, actually. I feel like a girl going on a date. I start to allow my anxieties and nervousness to give way to excitement. I push open the door, and walk towards the bar. I see Darren straight away, and he clocks me immediately, standing up and coming over to introduce himself. There is an embarrassing moment where he goes in for a kiss and I go to put my hand out and shake his, and I almost stab him in the stomach, but it's all OK in the end. He buys me a drink and we head over to a far table to get to know one another.

First impressions are good. He is a little older than he looks in his pictures, but that's okay. He looks more or less as I expected him to.

He's wearing a white shirt and cream chinos and throws his navy jumper over the back of his chair. He hands me my white wine and soda and smiles as I put it down on the table in front of me.

"Thank you," I say, and he lifts his glass to toast me.

"Lovely to meet you," he says, and we touch our glasses lightly together. When he smiles, I notice that he has good teeth. He doesn't have very nice eyes, though. Which is a bit of a shame, because I always think that nice eyes are a sign of a decent guy.

"So, tell me a little bit about yourself," he says. And, we are off...

We are doing the internet dating thing, revealing details about ourselves which will help us work out whether we want to spend time together, trying to work out whether there's a spark, trying to find areas of mutual interest.

The conversation flows nicely between us, with him chatting away, and we're discovering lots of people we think we might have in common. He lives in Esher, which is where my mum and dad live, I'm not far away in Cobham. He's been to the DIY and gardening shop where I work and tells me what fun it was in there at Christmas. I was the one put in charge of Christmas, so I feel a warm glow of appreciation at this comment.

"So, what's your dating history then?" I say, and he tells me that his most recent girlfriend dumped him just a couple of weeks ago. He looks absolutely heartbroken as he says this, and a little red flag pops up in my mind. The first red flag, so nothing to be too scared about.

"Had you been seeing her long?" I ask.

"No," he says. "Not a long time, and we had only been on a handful of dates, but when she disappeared suddenly without contacting me it brought back all sorts of terrible memories..."

Ah, I think to myself, ghosting. I remember Juan telling me about that. I don't share the news with Darren that this is a very common thing in the world of internet dating, though.

"The memories..." Darren is saying.

"Is everything all right?" I ask. I'm not sure whether I'm supposed to ask any more detail about his personal life or let him sit there, drifting back into memories.

"My wife died ten years ago," he says. "She was the love of

my life, I adored her. She was everything to me. I hadn't dated since her death, I concentrated on bringing up our daughter, then I decided to make room for dating, and I went out and met Marissa, but then she just disappeared. No explanation, no word about why she didn't want to see me again. Just gone.

"The whole incident has brought back the pain of losing my wife. It's been a tricky couple of weeks, to be honest."

"Goodness," I say. "Losing your wife like that must've been terrible."

"It was horrific," he says. "She was a teacher at a local junior school, and after we had our baby - Susie - she went in to show the teachers our new little girl. When she walked out, pushing our baby in a pushchair, a motor bike swerved off the road crashed into her and killed her. He missed Susie by inches."

"Gosh," I say, my hand flying up to my mouth and my eyes wide in disbelief. "That must've been absolutely awful."

"She was in a coma for a week, then I had to switch off the machine," he says. "Awful doesn't begin to cover it."

"I'm so, so sorry," I keep repeating, in the absence of words that better sum up the way I'm feeling. What do you say to a complete stranger when he starts revealing this sort of thing to you?

"Do you mind if we head back soon?" he says, after a short silence. "I really like you but I'm afraid I'm not going to give a very good account of myself. I'll just get more and more upset if we stay here like this. Maybe I can see you another time when I'm not feeling so awful?"

"Of course, that's no problem at all," I say, reaching for my bag. "There is a bus due in five minutes. I'll head off now and jump on it."

"Absolutely not," says Darren. "I wouldn't hear of it. Please,

Cobham is about five minutes away, let me drop you at home, it's the least I can do."

"If you're sure," I say.

"I'm absolutely sure," he says, standing up. "I'm very sorry about tonight...I don't know why I suddenly got so maudlin. I'm normally quite good company, or so I'm told."

"Please don't worry, it's not a problem at all," I say as I follow him outside and climb into his car next to him.

In truth, I'm not at all bothered about tonight. He seems like a nice chap, but there was certainly no spark between us, and he's got a long way to go to start feeling better about himself again before he can really date anyone properly.

He pulls out from the curb, and drives towards the end of the road, approaching a roundabout at which he has to turn left. But he indicates right and goes all the way round the roundabout. I suddenly have a panic in the pit of my stomach. Why is he not taking me home?

I've given him my address; he knows this is the wrong way.

"This isn't the way to go," I say, slightly nervously.

"Yes, I know," he says. "Will you just bear with me? There's something I really want to show you."

"Of course," I say. "Will it take very long?"

"Nope, we're just here." He pulls over to the side of the road and puts on his hazard warning lights. "Here," he says.

"Here?" I repeat. "Why have you brought me here?"

"This is where she was hit by the motorcycle. Right here, in that spot. Her body was lying across the road there. There was blood everywhere. The ambulance and police cars came that way, and parked there. I ran over and tried to hold her and talk to her. I lay next to her and was covered in her blood. The blood really was everywhere. Then they took her to hospital."

I just look at him. I don't know what to say, or do. He is staring at the road, but in his mind, he is back ten years, to when his life suddenly spun off its axis.

"I'd like to go home now," I say, and he drives off, taking me home without either of us saying another word.

SECOND DATE: STUART

Juan and Charlie sit on the sofa in stunned silence, while Dave paces around the room, punching his fist into his hand.

"What a dick," he says.

"No, no, he's not a dick. He's just still grieving. I guess his girlfriend disappearing brought back all the memories of losing his wife."

"I don't care how upset he was, you don't take someone on a first date to see where your wife was crushed by a motorbike," says Dave.

"And without telling you. If he'd said that he wanted to visit the place where his wife died, and would you like to come, you could have said 'no thanks, you giant weirdo, I want to go home'. But not to ask you, and to assume that you might actually want to go? On a first date? The man's a freak."

"We are coming with you tomorrow night," said Charlie.

"We will sit either in a nearby pub so you can reach us in an emergency or in the pub itself."

"No, that's crazy. There's no need. Look, I've obviously made this guy sound odder that he was. He was actually really nice."

"No!" says Dave. "No, no. He was odd. He showed you where the blood splatters were on the road when his wife was killed. If you don't think that's odd and very inappropriate, you need to have much higher standards."

"And where are your necklaces?" asks Juan. "Did he steal your necklaces?"

"What?" says Dave. "He stole from you?"

"No, he did nothing of the kind. They are in my bag. I'm fine. Please - all of you stop making this into a drama. I'm going to bed."

"*It is a drama*!" they all call after me.

Next day, I'm up early and off to work, leaving Juan in the flat.

Charlie's also at work today so he's all alone and God only knows what mischief he'll get up to. I've told him he must not go down and bother Dave all day.

"I won't," he says.

"You won't accidentally get locked out wearing nothing but a pink G-string?"

"Ooooo...stop putting ideas in my mind."

"Juan!"

"No, I promise I won't."

"OK then."

In the end he seems to have spent most of the day staking out the pub I'm meeting tonight's date in, and working out where he and Charlie could place themselves out of sight, but able to pounce if the date goes wrong. By the time I get back that evening he's planned it like a military invasion.

He has a detailed map of the pub garden printed out.

"We will enter from this direction," he says, showing me red arrows drawn onto the map. "This is the likely rendezvous point."

He shows a purple squiggle that he's drawn next to the bar. "So, you two will probably sit here..." There's another squiggle (green) drawn at a table near the bar.

"Perfect," I say. "Now I'm going to get changed because I'm meeting him in an hour."

"I've laid out your clothes on your bed," he says.

"What? Am I not allowed to make any decisions myself?"

"None," says Juan.

I go into my room to see that, happily, he's put out black trousers and high boots for tonight. It's chillier this evening than it was yesterday, and it's bound to get cold as the evening goes on, especially if we're outside. I put away the frilly top that he made me buy and pull out the loose-fitting cream jumper that I like and which actually fits me (the frilly blouse strains across my chest, which Juan seems to think is a good thing, but I most definitely do not).

I emerge from the room and stand there, ready for his inspection.

"More make-up," insists Juan, sending me back to my room to put on the brightest lipstick I own. I come back out and am greeted by a frown.

"This is it," I say. "This is as much make-up as I can bear to put on."

"What about the frilly blouse?"

I tell him that I'm wearing it under the jumper (a damn lie), and we head for the pub. When we arrive, Juan tells me to act normally, as if the two of them weren't there, and they would leap into action if things get difficult.

There is huge comedy potential in this scenario, though I don't mention it to Juan who is being such a sweetheart, insisting on coming with me. But the thought of Charlie and Juan leaping into action and beating up a badly-behaved suitor is a very strange thought. Together, they weigh less than I do. I can't imagine Charlie ever fighting with anyone, she is the most gentle and lovely person ever, and I don't imagine Juan is a secret Mike Tyson - though he was awesome in that dress shop. Let's just hope that back-up is not required.

I go into the pub to get myself a glass of wine from the bar then head back outside, sitting down at the loveliest table I can find, one that allows me to catch the last of the day's rays while being able to see Charlie and Juan on the other side of the beer garden. Juan is waving wildly. I thought they were supposed to be undercover over there?

Charlie nudges him as if reading my mind, and he lowers his hands slowly.

I take a large sip and sit back in my chair. I can't work out whether to wear my sunglasses or not. I'm never really sure whether they make me look mysterious and elegant or simply unapproachable and daft?

I'm doing the ridiculous on, off, on again with the glasses when a man appears in the garden and looks around. He fits the brief that's been given to me by Charlie and Juan but doesn't seem to be coming over to me. When I look over at them, they are smiling and putting the thumbs up, this is clearly him. He is a nice-looking man, stocky but not fat, quite big and manly looking. Very attractive, in fact. I pull the sunglasses off and smile over at him. He stops in his tracks and looks back. Then he walks into the bar, clearly not recognising that it's me. What do I do now? Run after him? I decide to sit there for a couple of minutes while he gets his drink, and he might wander back out again when he sees I'm not in the bar. So, I sit back, take another gulp of wine, and smile over at Charlie.

Just as I'm relaxing, a shadow is cast over me, and I look up to see the man who was in the garden earlier.

"Ah, hello. You must be Stuart?" I say, standing up. He's very attractive close up. "I'm Mary."

"Oh, it is you...I wasn't sure," he mutters, taking two enormous gulps of his drink.

"I know, it's hard, isn't it? When you don't quite know who you're looking for. Nice to meet you."

I put out my hand and he looks at it as if I've pulled a knife on him.

He's just staring at it. Then he takes another huge gulp of his drink and plonks his glass down heavily, causing the small metal table to shake a little on the unsteady ground, and some of the beer to splash out of the top and onto my cream jumper.

"Look, I can't do this," he says. "I'm really sorry. I'm sure you're lovely. But this isn't going to work for me." Then he backs away leaving me standing there with splashes of beer on my jumper. I see Charlie and Juan getting to their feet.

"I'm sorry...you're fatter than I thought you'd be. I'm sorry. That sounds rude but - well - you're too fat for me. I am very, very sorry."

By now, Juan has reached us.

"Sorry?" he says. "You're 'very, very sorry'? You dog."

Stuart looks alarmed by the arrival of Juan and the lecture he's getting, so he just runs. I've never seen anything like it. He sprints off through the garden towards the carpark as if he's being chased by lions. Juan runs after him, hurling expletives in Spanish.

"Eres horrible, feo, cerdo," he cries. "Cómo puedes tratar a mi amigo así?"

Charlie and I watch him go. We have no idea what he's shouting, but we know it's not pleasant.

"Mary es bella," he shouts at Stuart's retreating back. "Mary es bella."

Then he turns around and walks back to us. "Pig," he says. "You are too good for that little pig."

Juan gives me a big hug. "Who does he think he is? Running away like that. Does he think he's Usain Bolt or something? Pig. Now, we get drunk." Juan leads me to the bar, with Charlie in hot pursuit.

"Now we get very drunk and forget all about Dead Wife Darren last night and Usain Bolt this night. There are better men to come, Mary. I promise you; better men are out there."

After that we do drink a lot, to be fair – we consume vast amounts of alcohol, but I do that thing where I feel more and more sober, the more I drink. I'm not desperately unhappy or anything. Surprisingly it doesn't bother me what the guy said. This whole dating lark is showing me that I'm much more resilient than I ever thought I was.

Usain Bolt can say what he wants. I know I'm fat, for God's sake. Does he think I don't have mirrors? And I'd love to lose weight, but right now I'm this weight, and if the fact that I like cake is such a deal breaker for him, then we probably weren't going to get on anyway.

The only thing that I do feel slightly miserable about is the fact that every failed dating experience makes me think about

Ted and how amazingly perfect he was. I thought I was going to spend the rest of my life with Ted. It makes me so sad that I'm not, and am now going on dates with all these strange guys. Why the hell did it all go wrong? Perhaps I should call him and make it up to him?

"Hi," says a slurred voice, as I sit there, phone in hand, wondering whether to call.

"Hello," I reply. "I'm not very good company at the moment."

"I'll be the judge of that," he says, dropping into a seat next to me and raising his glass. I lift mine too and gently clink it against his. "I'm Harry."

"I'm Mary," I reply.

"I saw what happened," he says. "Earlier. You know - the idiot running off."

"Yeah - that wasn't great," I reply.

"He's a dick."

"No - I think you'll find he's a pig," I reply, and we both collapse into laughter.

"Yes. The sight of your friend running after him, screaming at him in a foreign language made my night."

"At least it turned a nasty evening into a very funny one."

"Don't think of it as a nasty evening," says Harry. "Think of him as a nasty person, but also think of the lovely friends who stood up for you and think of me - someone who has met you and really likes you."

"You really like me? But you don't know me."

"I've been listening to you and your friends talk. You seem lovely."

"Thank you," I say.

"Would you come out for a drink with me one night, you know – just to get to know one another better?"

"Really?"

"Yes, really. Maybe tomorrow night?"

"I'm not sure whether I'm free tomorrow," I say. "Can I text you and let you know?"

"Of course," he says, and he puts his number into my phone.

I smile to myself at how funny it is that I have to consult the dating programme before I know when I can fit him in. I may be on the wrong side of 25 and several pounds overweight, but this dating lark might be turning out OK after all.

Later that night, having explained that I'd like to squeeze another date into the programme, I sit next to Charlie while she looks through the timetable.

"You know this is going to cause all sorts of administrative problems for me, don't you?" she says, as she deploys pencils, rubbers and rulers to her rather complicated-looking chart. "I'll have to adjust everyone, and we'll have to take someone out if you want to add the new guy in."

"Wouldn't it be funny," I say. "If, after all the work you've done to try and introduce me to new men, I end up dating someone I bumped into myself."

"Funny? I can think of other words for it – like bloody annoying," says Charlie.

"You love me, really," I say, reaching over to give her a hug, but I'm not as sure-footed as I thought I was, and I stumble into her, almost flattening her. Perhaps I'm drunker than I realised.

"Yes – I love you really," she says, her voice coming up from somewhere beneath me. "Now get off me and let me see whether I can make this work."

"Perfect," I say. "Now, I better go to bed."

THIRD DATE: MARTIN

I feel quite conspicuous walking up the street towards the Post Office at 5.30pm to meet tonight's date. It's quite an odd place to meet someone - the Post Office - and this is so early. But he insists that there's a lovely café nearby that we can go to, and that earlier is better. Charlie and Juan have parked themselves in the pub opposite so they are nearby in case anything happens. After last night's runaway date, Juan is keener than ever to make sure that he is nearby in case there are any problems. I've let them come tonight, but I've decided to stop them coming to the rest of the dates, or it will get crazy.

As I approach the Post Office, I can see that my date is not there yet, there is just a guy with his young kid, looking at all the postcards on the noticeboard. So, I stop at the furniture shop next door which has a big mirror in the window, and adjust my hair. I am pouting and preening and double-checking there is no lipstick on my teeth when I feel a gentle tap on my shoulder.

"Are you Mary?" says the guy with the young boy.

"Yes."

"I'm Martin. Lovely to meet you." He puts his hand out to shake mine. This is so weird. Why's he got a kid with him?

"Can I introduce Matt?"

Matt is about five years old, and looks like he'd rather be anywhere else on Earth than meeting me.

"Hello Matt," I say, as the little boy looks at the ground and digs his hands in his pockets.

"Don't be rude, shake the nice lady's hand," says Martin. Matt just looks up at me from beneath a floppy fringe and sneers a little.

"Don't worry," I say quickly. "It's lovely to meet you, Matt."

"I hope you didn't mind meeting at the Post Office. It seemed the easiest place. I thought we could go to the café at the end of the road for a bite to eat. They do half price kids' meals on Thursdays."

"Sure," I say. I'm not quite sure whether this is some sort of joke. I don't mean to be rude, and it must be hard to find babysitters and all that, but who in God's name brings their child on a date with them?

We head to the café at the corner of the road, with Martin spending the whole time telling Matt to stop fiddling with his hair, and to put away his electronic game. Matt doesn't utter a sound, not even a grunt. We get to the café and Martin goes in first, and orders a table for two before adding quickly, "Oh no, sorry, no – a table for three. Sorry, I forgot Mary was with us."

Forgot Mary was with us? Forgot Mary was with us? This is supposed to be a date that you're on *with Mary*.

We sit down at our table which is next to lots of other tables, forming a circle around a play area in the middle. Matt rushes into the play area, and shrieks along with the other children as they do that game you find in every doctor's waiting room, where you have to slide the coloured balls around twisting metal poles.

I look down at the table with its grubby, Formica tablecloth. There are crayons and papers on it for the children, and a 'design a hat' competition. Martin smiles at the adults there. They are clearly parents from Matt's school. Christ, it was bad enough when I thought he'd brought Matt on his evening out with me, but now I realise he's brought me on his evening out with Matt. This is crackers. He chats to the other parents who are there (mainly mums), but doesn't introduce me, so I sit in silence while they discuss some forthcoming school trip.

"I used to love school trips when I was little," I say. "They were always good fun."

"Do you have children?" asks one of the mothers sitting opposite.

She's very attractive - slim and elegant, with a blonde bob, skinny jeans and a floaty green blouse.

"No, I don't," I say, and she turns back and carries on with what she was doing.

This is ridiculous. I'm not quite sure what to do or what to say.

Should I just walk out? But then the waitress arrives and takes our order. I order orange squash with fish fingers and chips because that's what everyone else seems to be ordering. Then I head off to the toilets which smell strongly of nappies. Each cubicle has a small potty in it. I sink down onto the toilet seat, pulling my phone out to text Juan.

"Reinforcements required. I seem to be on a play date with a bunch of five-year-olds. I'm at the café on the corner of High Street and Station Road. Please help!"

I look at myself in the mirror, all dressed up, hair freshly styled, wearing my new earrings and favourite lipstick. I look better than I have for ages, all to sit in a café with a bunch of children.

Back in the café I discover a scrawny little boy has climbed into my seat. His skinny legs protrude from oversized shorts. "Do you want to play action man with me?" he asks.

"Of course she does," says Martin. He turns to me. "You'd like that, wouldn't you?"

My phone bleeps in my bag and I pray with all my might that it's Juan confirming that they are on their way.

"Of course I would," I tell the boy, and I pick up a broken action man and dress him as a soldier, while other children gather round and join in the fun.

"We need more soldiers," shouts a sandy-haired boy. "Bring all of the action men over here."

The action men are duly brought over, along with all the children.

"Now we can do a proper war," says sandy-haired boy to Skinny Legs.

"Come on," he says to me. "Bring your man out."

I'm just marching my one-legged Action Man into war when the little bell on the door rings, and the extravagant Juan and gorgeous Charlie walk into the café and stop, open-mouthed, as they see me and dozens of five-year-olds playing wargames with action men.

"What on earth?" says Charlie, as skinny legs tells me to surrender.

The others all jump up and down screaming "surrender," so I drop my action man on his back.

"I surrender," I say. "But I thought we were all on the same side."

"Of course not," says Sandy Hair.

Charlie and Juan have made their way through the café and are standing next to me.

Juan says something in Spanish which probably wouldn't bear translating in front of the all the children, and I shrug my shoulders.

"You've beaten me," I say to Skinny Legs. "Now you're king of all the world."

"That's not how it works," replies Skinny Legs. "You don't become king of all the world just because you win a fight."

"Well, you should," I say.

Then I turn to Martin. "I'm afraid I have to go, something's come up," I say, standing up and bidding farewell to everyone.

"Oh no, you're not going, are you? I like you a lot. Please stay," comes a voice. But it's not the voice of Martin, who couldn't give a toss whether I'm there or not. It's the voice of the little boy with the skinny legs.

"I'm so sorry," I say. "But I have to go to work now. I'll tell you what – you can have my fish fingers when they come."

"Yum!" says the boy. And I head towards the door, while all the parents look at me in complete confusion. They don't know why I came, and they have no idea why I'm suddenly leaving.

Just as I'm almost through the door, Skinny Legs comes charging towards me and grabs me, begging me to stay.

"Shoo, shoo," says Juan, attempting to move the kid from me in the way one might dispense pigeons landing on the table. "Shoo, shoo," he repeats.

Eventually one of the mothers comes over and takes her son back.

He bursts into tears when I wave at him. Martin, meanwhile, doesn't seem to have looked up from his colouring book.

BALLS ON SHOW

It's my date with Harry today – the guy I met in the pub after the Usain Bolt disaster. I've been looking forward to this one, and was planning to spend the day relaxing and beautifying myself so I look as good as possible. But there's no chance to relax as I'm dragged, cruelly, from my slumber by the sound of a commotion outside the window. Raised voices and a car revving maniacally outside wrest me from my sleep. What fresh hell is this? I pull back the curtains and peer through. Down below I see Dawn standing by her car, hands on hips, while a guy sits in the driver's seat revving it.

Shit, I completely forgot that Dawn was coming today. She's an old school friend who I became reacquainted with recently when she came into the shop, announced that she ran a travel blog, and promptly invited me to come on safari with her. Free! I went swiftly from barely recognising her, to declaring that she was the best friend I'd ever had. I've been on a few more trips for her blog since then, and though Dawn isn't exactly my cup of tea (she can be very aggressive), she's been kind and generous to me over the years.

I jump away from the window, pull the curtains closed and run around getting myself dressed and looking half decent. I rush into the living room where Juan Pedro is standing, one leg extended behind him in an arabesque.

"Morning, darling, just doing my wake-up exercises," he says, before swinging his leg round and holding it out in front in such an elegant way that I feel moved to stop and watch him for a while. I have no idea how he does that.

"I think Dawn is here," he says. "But I'm staying away because it sounds like they're having car trouble and are getting very aggressive out there. Cars and aggression are two things I don't do."

"Yes, I heard all the shouting and the engine revving... I suppose I better go out and check everything is OK."

Juan brings his leg down to the floor and turns with a flourish to follow me out of the flat. "I'm coming as back-up," he says. "But I'm not touching any engines...or any oily big ends."

We get outside to hear Dawn bellowing at her boyfriend, Steve. He is a rough-looking chap with more tattoos than hair, and the sort of gruff voice that can only be earned by regularly inhaling smoke. The man must be on about 80 cigarettes a day.

"Darling Mary, how are you?" says Dawn when she sees me, dropping her argument with Steve as she moves to embrace me.

"Let me introduce Juan," I say, indicating Juan standing next to me.

Dawn's eyes open wide as she takes in his attire... Very baggy harem trousers that make him look a bit like Aladdin, and a tight gold T-shirt. It's funny, I get used to the way Juan dresses, so it doesn't surprise me to see him looking like someone in a pantomime. But the looks of other people remind me that he has a very original take on fashion.

"I'm going to have to go under the car, love," says Steve. He climbs out of the driver's seat and I see that he is wearing quite small shorts for a large man. I have to stop my gaze dropping to his shorts area.

"Nice to see you," I say. "My name is Mary."

"Steve," he says, kissing me on the cheek. Then turns to look Juan up and down. "You must be Ted."

"I'm Juan," he says, quickly. "I'm a friend of Mary's."

"Right, let's get this thing up in the air and have a look what's going on, shall we?" he says, taking a jack out of the boot and beginning to lift the front of the car. He messes around for a while stabilising it, then eases himself underneath it, until just his legs and his shorts are sticking out.

"Have you got a torch?" he says. "And maybe some rags or something?"

"Sure, I'll go and have a look now," I say, heading back into my flat.

Dawn follows me and we rummage around until we have found everything he needs. Then we head back outside. Dawn reaches down to hand the rags to Steve, with me by her side. But as she reaches out to him, she sees that he's popped right out of his shorts.

I see it too. His testicles are a most alarming sight.

"Oh my God," she says, dropping the rags and leaning over to tuck him back inside. In doing so she reaches right into his shorts, giving him a quick fondle and giggling to herself. Then she rearranges the shorts to make sure he doesn't escape again, cupping him to make sure he's all tucked up inside. After giving him the rags and the torch, she stands up. I stand next to her. Standing next to us is…Steve. He is staring at her as if she's lost her mind.

"Who the hell is under that car?" says Dawn. We both look down at the pavement at the man she's just fondled. Then the man pushes himself back. It's Dave.

"What the hell was that?" he says.

"I thought you were my boyfriend," says Dawn.

"No. No, I'm not," he replies.

"I can see that now," says a red-faced Dawn.

"Dave came out and offered to help, so he is sorting out the oil leak," says Juan.

Steve says nothing… He just stares at Dawn like he can't believe what she just did. To be honest, none of us can quite believe what she just did, least of all Dawn herself. Dave has turned the brightest pink imaginable and won't meet anyone's eyes.

"I think you'd better come inside," I say to Dawn and Steve. "Let's have a nice cup of tea." We all chat amiably for a little while without anyone mentioning what Dawn just did.

"The reason I wanted to come and see you," she says, when she's regained the power of speech. "Is that I've got lots of trips on the go at the moment, if you fancy going on any of them."

"Oh my God, I'd love to go off on holiday somewhere. "Is it for the blog?"

"Yes. And you can take someone. If there are any hot men in your life right now, tell them they can come on a trip with you. Call me and I'll fix it up straight away. You just have to remember to report back on the blog four times a day, and send videos and pictures."

"Yes, that's not a problem," I say, thinking of a dreamy holiday somewhere, and how amazing that would be.

"Thanks so much, Dawn," I say. "That's brilliant."

With that, she's off. Most peculiar. I appreciate her coming over here to tell me I can go on a free holiday if I like, and I'm sure Dave appreciated the quick fondle, but there's something a bit odd about it all…

FOURTH DATE: NO HARRY

I am still mulling over Dawn's visit while I prepare to head out that evening to meet Harry. My plans to spend the day relaxing and beautifying were blown to smithereens by the visit from Dawn offering me the chance to go on more holidays. Where will I end up? Somewhere romantic like St Lucia, perhaps? I've always really fancied going there. Have you seen it? It's all turquoise oceans and beaches fringed with palm trees, white sands and boats with white sails. I've never seen anywhere so beautiful before.

Or somewhere romantic like Italy? Anywhere, really. I just love the thought of going away.

My warming thoughts are broken by the ringing of my phone. It is Harry.

"Hello."

"It's Harry here. You're going to hate me."

"Am I?"

"Yes, look I can't make it tonight."

"Great," I reply sarcastically, before I can stop myself.

"I'm sorry," he says.

"Don't worry. It's better than you coming then running away. At least you've had the decency to phone."

"It's my mum," he says. "She's really ill. I'm in hospital with her."

"Oh. Gosh. Is she OK?"

"A small heart attack, she should be OK, though. I just don't want to leave her while she's feeling so weak and scared."

"No, I completely understand. Go and see her, and thanks for letting me know."

I put the phone down and there's a text straight away. It's from Dave, wishing me luck on my date.

"He's cancelled," I reply. "His mum is in hospital."

"Oh really," says Dave. "Did he suggest another date?"

"No," I say.

"Then he could be benching you."

Great. Thanks, Dave.

FIFTH DATE: RUPERT

I wake up to a text from Harry, asking me whether we can meet soon.

"OK," I say, though I know Charlie won't be happy that she has to change the timetable again. She's very inflexible with her dating diary.

"I'll let you know when I can make it. How's your mum?"

"She's not great, but she's in the right hands. I told her all about you."

"Did you?" I say. "That's really nice."

"Well, you're really nice. You'll call me soon and let me know when we can catch up, won't you?"

"Yes," I reply, feeling a little bit light-headed. Dave is wrong; I'm not being benched. Harry's a really nice guy.

I'm off work today, so I'm going to get my nails done, and my eyebrows waxed before tonight's date. That is how committed I am to this process!

Since I'm going to be wearing cream tonight (yes – the same

dress again....I hope these daters never meet and discuss my attire), I have decided to get my nails painted in a gorgeous fudge colour. I know that sounds horrid, but it looks great on the model in the beauticians so I decide to give it a try. I'm pleased to say that it works well, and as I lay back on the bed to have my eyebrows waxed into shape, I look at them admiringly.

"OK then. What sort of thing were you thinking of?" says Melody the stylist, sizing up my eyebrows as she pushes and pulls them, lifts them and separates them. "They are quite bushy. Shall I give them a whole new shape?"

"I'm not sure," I say.

"I just think it would look a bit more modern."

"I thought the rage was for bigger eyebrows?"

"Yes, but not quite this big."

"OK, fine," I say. "You do what you think is best."

Then I lay back and think of people with perfect eyebrows, like Meghan Markle and Cheryl Cole.

TWO HOURS LATER...

"It's not that bad," say Juan and Charlie.

"It looks painful, though," Charlie adds. "Does it hurt?"

"Of course it hurts," I say. "It stings and feels raw. And obviously I look as if I've been rubbing my face up against sandpaper. This bloke I'm going on a date with tonight is going to think I'm a nutter."

"He might not," says Juan. "Some people are into that sort of thing. I met this guy once who said he went to a gay orgy and one of the guys pulled out really rough sandpaper..."

"Okay, okay, not helping," I cry.

I don't need to hear from Juan that the only people likely to be interested in me are those who prefer vigorous sex involving sandpaper.

"What am I going to do?"

Besides the fact that my face looks red raw in a streak along my eyebrows, there's also the fact that my eyebrows have been so overly shaped that there is hardly anything left of them and I look really peculiar.

"Did you say anything to her?" says Charlie. "You know, like tell her she stripped off your skin and made you look ridiculous."

"No, of course I didn't," I reply. "I'm British. I never complain about anything. I just wanted to get out of there as quickly as possible and head home."

"Was it the same place you had that facial before, where you looked like you'd been boiled alive for a couple of days?"

"Err, yes," I say. I know I shouldn't have gone back there, but it's so much cheaper than everywhere else.

"Do you think I look OK, Juan?" I say.

"Well, you look like a burns victim," he says, with a distinct lack of consideration for my feelings. "But this is what makeup was made for. We will get you fixed up and looking glorious in no time at all."

Half an hour later…

I don't look glorious. I should say that right at the start. I've got so much make-up on I look like a bloody geisha girl.

"You just look perfectly made up, and as if you've made an effort," says Charlie, in an attempt to reassure me.

"Yes, I've made an effort for someone who wants to be a clown."

"I didn't know what else to do," says Juan. "I thought I would put make-up on just around the eyebrows, but I didn't realise how much I had to put, and then it looked very odd with the rest of the face, so I had to put it on the rest of the face as well, and – well – this is the result."

"You look lovely, please don't worry," says Charlie.

They are both standing in the hallway, looking at me as I look at myself in the mirror. To be fair to Juan, he's done a good job. I look a lot better than I did earlier. You can't see the lightning streaks of raw red around my eyes, and my eyebrows are now back to a normal shape. Much fuller than they were a few hours earlier thanks to Juan's artistic flair with pencils and brushes. There's nothing wrong with what he's done, it's just that there's way too much of it. Honestly, I must have half a bottle of foundation on my face.

"Just don't rub your eyebrows, because they're 90% eyeliner pencil," says Juan. "Then you'll be okay."

"OK," I say. "I guess I should go and meet this guy…"

I have managed to persuade Charlie and Juan not to come with me on this date…it's in a small, cozy pub, and it will be obvious that they are there.

"I'll be fine," I promise them. "I'll text you when I'm leaving."

The only thing I know about Rupert is that he is 42 (but he looks a lot older than that in his picture). He looks nice, and Charlie's notes on him say that he is very courteous, well-spoken and obviously quite bright and well off, which augurs well.

We've arranged to meet at a bar near Hampton Court Palace.

It's a lovely place with tables outside from which you can see the palace on one side and the river on the other side. I think it might be my favourite pub in the whole world, called the Phoenix Arms. Inside it has a Baroque feel with loads of gorgeous big velvet armchairs and sofas in wonderful jewel colours, piles of cushions and gentle music on in the background. There is a small gin bar in one corner and the main bar serving all the usual drinks. Upstairs is a restaurant that offers the best views imaginable toward the palace. It is called, predictably enough, 'The Henry VIII'. We have arranged to meet downstairs, though Rupert suggested to Charlie that if I fancy dinner, we could do that afterwards.

I walk into the bar and don't see him at first. He is tucked in a corner of the room, folded into one of the big velvet sofas. I smile to myself as I see him clambering out of it in a very ungainly fashion - he's all knees and elbows as he staggers to his feet. As I predicted, he's much older than his photo indicated. He looks strangely familiar, though I've no idea where I might know him from. Perhaps he just has one of those faces?

He has a lovely manner, and bounds up to me, smiling and proffering his hand, but he also hugs me into him and kisses me on the cheek.

"What can I get you to drink, then?" he says, with an impish smile and a Bambi-ish demeanor that makes me feel unaccountably happy.

"I'd love a gin and tonic, especially if they have any of those fruity flavours, like rhubarb. I love those."

"Oh, that does sound good, let's go over the gin bar and see what they've got."

This, I predict, is going to be a very successful date.

He is considerably older than me, and I wouldn't say I fancy him, as such, but then I didn't fancy Ted when I first met him. His personality was what won me over and make me feel great.

I'm sure the same thing could happen again, if I get to know this guy.

He certainly seems lovely. With a bit of luck, he won't have any dead wives or young children that he wants to introduce me to.

We take our drinks over to two beautiful green velvet armchairs.

"I think these chairs might be safer," he says. "It took me about 20 minutes to get out of that sofa over there. I wouldn't want to subject you to that."

I smile. I love his self-deprecating humour, and warmth.

As I look at him, he does seem really familiar.

"Do you live round here?" I ask him.

"Yes, I do," he says. "I live and work in the area. I do love Hampton Court."

"Me too," I say. "I don't come here anywhere near enough. Whenever I do come, I think how amazingly beautiful it is."

"We should go to the Palace for the day, one time," he says, all wide-eyed and friendly. "We could have a tour around and learn all about the wives, and the incredible tyrant who lived there."

"Oh yes, that would be fantastic," I say.

"So, tell me all about yourself," he says, and I talk about my job in the DIY centre, how I met Ted, and we got on brilliantly and had a lovely relationship, but it seemed to have run its course so we have gone our separate ways. He tells me that he used to be married too, but they split a long time ago and his wife remarried. He works as a locum doctor moving between practices, but he also has a private practice which is his main focus, and there he treats mainly children.

"I love it," he says. "It's very difficult treating children because they're not as good as adults are at expressing what's wrong, so you have to fiddle around and interpret what they're saying much more, but when you solve a child's problem it is the loveliest feeling in the world."

"I bet it is," I say. "It must be great to be able to make people better."

"Yes, I'm very lucky to have a job that I love so much."

I notice that his glass is already empty.

"Would you like another drink?" I ask.

"No, let me get this," he says, reaching down to his jacket that has fallen onto the floor, to pull out his wallet. He looks up at me. "Same again?"

That's when I realise where I know him from, as he looks up at me the memory comes flooding back. The last time I saw him he looked up at me like that…from between my legs…and I had no knickers on.

"I think I know where I know you from," I say, all hesitant and flushed with embarrassment. "Do you sometimes work as a gynaecologist?"

"Yes, I work in all areas of general practice. Is that a problem?"

"No, not a problem, but I think you worked as my gynaecologist. I came in to see you earlier in the week. I lost my knickers."

It's all too weird for words. I just can't cope with this. This guy is my gynaecologist. How can I sit and have a drink with him? I feel so embarrassed, though he seems entirely unperturbed. He stands to go over to get the drinks while I drop my head into my hands, running them through my hair and across my face. Trying to calm myself down and work out what to do.

He arrives back and his eyes almost pop out of his head.

"Your eyebrows have completely disappeared," he says. "And

you've got soot or something all over your forehead. Are you OK?"

"Oh Christ, that's my eyebrows," I say. "I was rubbing my face. Oh, never mind."

I can't sit here and have a drink with a guy who had his hand inside me just a few days previously. It's no good at all.

"I'm so sorry," I say. "You seem like a really top man, but you're my gynaecologist. This is so weird. Do you mind if I leave?"

"Goodness, I've just bought the drinks," he says. "Are you sure?"

"Yes, perfectly sure," I say, grabbing my handbag and my cardigan. "I'm really sorry. This is just making me feel so weird. I'm sorry."

I start to walk away and he calls after me.

"I found them, by the way," he says, standing up and shouting.

"Found what?"

"Your knickers," he says. "After you left, I found your knickers under the bed."

"Oh God," I say, and I run through the pretty pub, past the colourful sofas and the people at the bar who are now staring at me.

I can never, ever go back to that place again, and I can never, ever visit a gynaecologist again. EVER.

SIXTH DATE: HARRY (TAKE II)

"Nooooooo…" says Juan. "The very doctor who did your girly bits? He was the guy on the date?"

"YES!"

"Oh...it's too much!" Juan paces around the bedroom. To his credit, he's not laughing at the comic elements of this latest romantic fiasco, but appears to fully understand the awfulness of what happened.

"When did you realise who he was? As soon as he walked in?"

"No, it was when he looked up at me. It reminded me of when he looked up at me from between my legs."

"Oh Good Lord in heaven. I can't imagine. It's too much. But your date tonight will be nice. You know him and you know he is a lovely man because he looked after his mother when she was ill, so that is good."

"You don't think he was benching me?"

"No, because now he has made a date with you. I am happy now that he is nice, and decent, and normal."

"Yes," I say. "I'm looking forward to it. He's normal and hasn't seen my vagina, so it'll be a pleasant change."

Juan shudders dramatically and leaves to let me get ready.

At 6pm I walk into the pub and see Harry sitting there, focusing intently on the newspaper in front of him, poised with pen in hand.

He looks so serious, clearly trying to think of a clue that is evading him.

"Good evening," I say. "Are you struggling?"

"Yes. It's Sudoku...drives me nuts. I've no idea why I put myself through it."

I take a seat opposite him and he puts down his paper. "Don't let me forget that, will you?" he says. "I hate it if I put it down and forget to take it with me. These are mine, as well." There's a pile of newspapers on the floor by his feet.

"Gosh, you love your Sudoku, don't you?"

"Listen," he replies. "I've got a proposal for you. I could go to the bar and get us a drink here or, I don't know whether you fancy it, but I made some supper for us earlier. I didn't want to put you off by inviting you to mine, so I thought we'd meet here and see what you thought, but it's all there, waiting for us if you've hungry?

"It's just chili con carne with rice and some cheesy garlic bread, and I've made a big salad too...and some rosemary roasted potatoes.

"Do you fancy coming back for supper in the garden? I've got some wine at home too...completely up to you. No pressure. The food won't go to waste, so only if you want to."

I look at him for a moment. I know I shouldn't go back to

his flat but he does seem perfectly normal. And he likes newspapers. Men who like newspapers are usually fairly sober, straightforward and decent human beings, aren't they? And the food sounds soooo good.

"Sure," I say. "I'd like that."

His house is near the pub; a short stroll down a lovely, tree-lined street. I'm wondering how on earth he has managed to afford one of these big, imposing houses when we turn into a side road flanked by less salubrious properties. They are still nice, but much smaller and more in keeping with what I was expecting. There's a block of flats at the far side of the cul-de-sac. "This is me," he says, opening the front door and allowing me to pass through into a lovely, bright, airy reception area.

"This is great," I say.

"Oh, thank you. I really like it here. Look..." He walks me across the reception area, to the huge window on the other side which looks out onto the river.

"Oh my God...river views!" I shriek. "I thought they were an urban myth...I didn't know they actually existed."

"Ha, ha," he replies. "Yes, we're lucky here - river views, a gym in the basement and tennis court outside. It's a fine place."

"Wow," I say. "That does sound lovely."

"Not that I use the gym. Or the river views."

I just smile at this, because I don't quite know what he means. 'Don't use the river views'? How odd is that? Little do I know that, at this precise moment, a big, red flag has just gone up. I don't see it, of course. Only with hindsight will the significance of this comment become clear.

"Shall we head inside and I'll find us a little spot to have supper?" he says.

"Sure," I reply, following him along a corridor and standing back as he opens his door. He pushes it open and tells me to follow him, as he leads me into the room. It's dark inside, and I bash my knee against something.

"Hang on, I'll put the light on now, so you can see where you're going."

I hear him bashing and crashing as he fights along the corridor, and then he flicks on the light switch. Light floods in, and I can see the place in all its glory. There are boxes and piles of newspapers everywhere. I mean, EVERYWHERE.

"Oh, have you just moved in?" I say.

"No, been here for five years."

"Right. Only ...all the boxes?"

"Yes, I know - they are everywhere...come through."

I push my way through into the sitting room.

"Oh my God," I say when I get in there. The place is absolutely full of junk. I mean, packed with junk. I can hardly get through the door...it's completely insane. Big piles of newspapers sit around all over the floor, there are black binbags full of cans, cartons and more newspapers. I just stand and stare. I have no idea where to go, where to sit, or why on earth this is happening to me.

"Where would you like me to go?" I say.

"Do you mind if we stand?" he says. "I've got all my cartons over there and I don't want us to disrupt them, and those newspapers are from 2016, so I need to keep those."

"Why do you need to keep them?" I ask. "I mean – why do you need to keep any of this stuff?"

"Because I love it," he says. "If you could just stand here for a bit, I'll go and get the food ready."

He removes his jacket and out of the pocket he takes a pile of cutlery.

"Cutlery is my favourite," he says, walking into the kitchen. I follow him, hoping there might be a chair in the kitchen where I can sit while he cooks, though why I don't just leave at this point is a mystery to me. I mean – how on earth can we come back from all this madness?

The kitchen is crazily packed, and has about 14 times as much as the average kitchen might have in it. On the counter there are eight bags of sugar, three of them open, five of them unopened. I watch as he opens the drawers, one of which is completely packed with spoons.

He squeezes in all the spoons that he must have acquired from the pub earlier, then he puts the forks into the fork drawer and opens up a vegetable drawer in which the top two racks are full of newspapers and the bottom rack is packed full of knives which tumble out when he opens it. He throws the knives in and shuts it then turns round and jumps a little when he sees me.

"What are you doing here?" he says. "I thought you'd be relaxing in the sitting room."

"I thought I'd come and see whether you needed any help with dinner?"

"You could set the table if you like," he says, moving over to the sink where he has to walk round a big bucket full of potato peelings, and washes his hands. I open the drawers I've just seen him putting cutlery into and take out two forks and two knives.

"What on earth are you doing?" he says.

"You asked me to lay the table…"

"Yes, but we don't use that cutlery. I like to keep that cutlery; I don't want to use it."

"Okay," I say. "Where is the cutlery that you like to use?"

"Well, if the truth be known, I don't like to use any of it. I like to keep the cutlery. I like it to be special. You can look in that carrier bag on the counter. We can use that, but please be careful with it."

I put my hand into the carrier bag and it's full of plastic knives and forks. Again, there are absolutely loads of them. I take out two knives and two forks.

"Not those," he says. "The plain ones. Those are quite rare."

"They're plastic forks, Harry. How rare can they be?"

He glares at me before substituting the ones I chose with marginally plainer ones that he has selected.

"Can you tell me where the loo is?" I ask. I think I'll go quickly before dinner.

"It's over there, with the blue door. But why didn't you go in the pub?" he says.

"Because I didn't need to go then."

"Would you mind walking back to the pub to go to the loo? There's not much room in mine."

"No, I'm not walking back to the pub - I'll go in this one," I say.

"No," shouts Harry, running after me, but it's too late. I open the door and around a hundred newspapers come tumbling out of the room.

"Oh no," he says. "Please don't touch anything. Just go to the pub if you need the loo."

That's when I think that this is nuts.

"I'm really sorry about this," I say. "But I really think I should get back, and not stay for supper. But it was lovely to see you again."

"Why?" he says. "What's the matter?"

"Well there's nowhere to sit or anything because of the boxes, and I don't want to have to go to the pub."

"So, you're going to storm out because I like boxes and newspapers?"

As he's talking, he's putting the plastic knives and forks back into the carrier bag and I see him visibly relax when the plastic cutlery is put away.

"Yes, I've got a bit of a headache and I've got work early in the morning, so I might head off. Sorry. Hope that's okay."

I walk to the door, past all the enormous bags full of stuff and the boxes piled high with assorted paraphernalia, pull the door open and turn to give him a kiss on the cheek.

"Sorry to be a bore," I say, before leaving, speed walking down the path.

That man needs some serious help.

MISSING TED

I get to the end of the road, out of sight of Harry's flat, and sigh with relief before calling an Uber. Luckily it comes in five minutes and I collapse into the back, and immediately call Ted.

It's not something I do consciously, or with a great deal of planning. I just find that I've called him before I know what I'm doing...it goes straight to answerphone and I leave a message. "Hi...it's me. I...I don't know why I'm calling. I just miss you. Been on the worst date ever. It was crazy. He was a hoarder. Kept thinking of you and how mad you'd think it was…there were boxes everywhere. And cutlery. He was mad about cutlery. Worst date ever, honestly…"

I hang up. I shouldn't really have told Ted that I was going off on dates, but I imagine him roaring with laughter when he hears about it, hugging me and telling me he wants me back and I never need to go on another date again. Tears spring into the corners of my eyes, then more, then more again, until I am sobbing like crazy.

"You OK, love?" asks the taxi driver nervously.

"Yes," I reply, blowing my nose in an unladylike fashion and doing a horrible snort.

My phone bleeps. A text. I grab it...dying to see what Ted has to say, but it is hoarder man. "Seems strange that you rushed off when we were getting along so well. So, I have a few boxes in my house. Since when is that a crime? No wonder you're single. If you apologise, I'd be happy to meet you again."

Then, a reply from Ted. "So glad you're going on lots of dates. It must be wonderful for you. Ted."

I'VE BLOWN IT. I'VE LOST HIM FOREVER.

SEVENTH DATE: OLLYVER

Today I'm going on a date with a guy called Ollyver. For some reason it is making me really cross that he spells the name 'Oliver' in such an odd way. Why shove an extra 'l' and a 'y' into the mix? It's silly but it's making me feel very angry. I know my antipathy towards him is caused in no small part by the fact that I'm sad about Ted. The man is the love of my life but he seems to hate me now. I'm such an idiot. Charlie says I should call him, but I don't want to give him the pleasure of insulting me any further.

So, here I am - approaching today's date with a big dollop of sadness stuck somewhere deep in the pit of my stomach.

I spot Ollyver standing at the corner of the street, looking out and smiling when he sees me…to be fair to him, he looks really nice.

Perhaps Ollyver with the oddly spelt name, won't be quite such a moron after all? I mean, it wasn't him who chose the spelling of the name, was it? Perhaps he just has peculiar parents. And – let's be honest – we all have those.

"I'm Mary," I say, as I get close to him.

"Yes, I know," he says, with a smile. "I'm Ollyver."

He's carrying a sort of doctor's bag which gives me a small scare. Not someone else who's seen me naked? But then I realise it's more of a large document case. He must have come straight from the office.

"Well, it's very nice to meet you," I say, and he smiles a warm and friendly smile.

"There is a delicatessen on the corner here which has lovely food and great coffee if you fancy it?" he says. "Then we could go for a drink if you want. But I can't be late back because of my pets."

"Right, OK, well the delicatessen sounds good."

I'm torn between thinking that it's weird for him to announce that he has to rush back for his pets, and thinking that it's actually quite cool that he is looking after his pets properly. Presumably he has a dog that needs walking. If he's been out at work all day, it's only right that he should walk it in the evening.

The delicatessen is lovely, as he said it would be. It is all wooden but with white sparkly fairy lights all around the room, lighting up shelves that are covered with white ornaments, making it look clean and modern but also quite funky and original.

"I really like this," I say.

Actually, I should say that one of the nice things about doing this internet dating has been not only meeting a pile of new men, but also going to lots of places that I would never have gone to before. This delicatessen is only a couple of miles from my home, but I've never been here. I suppose going out and meeting new people does force you to go to new places, which isn't a bad thing at all.

We decide to order their 'special cream tea' which involves not just delicious scones, home-made jam and clotted cream, but a range of sandwiches and home-made cakes. It all sounds completely lovely.

While we're waiting for our tea to arrive, I chat to Ollyver about my day job. I've got a summary of it off pat now having regaled numerous suitors with the story of my life over the past few days.

Ollyver explains that he works in a factory, and is hoping to cut down his hours because he doesn't like the impact of his long hours on his pets. Once again, I have a feeling of being torn between thinking this is quite odd, and thinking it is quite nice to love your dog.

Our food comes on those cake stands that sit one on top of the other, with sandwiches on the bottom, a mixture of really delicious looking cakes on the next and scones on the top with pots of jam and clotted cream.

"Enjoy," says the lady who delivers them. She has flour on her apron and looks as if she has come straight from the kitchen where she's been baking all afternoon. This is such a homely place but with an artistic, contemporary feel. I've fallen in love with it slightly more than I have with Ollyver. He is very nice, but we don't have a great deal in common, and not being a pet owner myself, I don't think I can really chat as much as he wants to about the trials and tribulations of looking after animals.

I take a big bite out of one of the sandwiches and notice that Ollyver is tearing bits of his sandwich off so he has a pile of little bits on his plate. Then he takes some of the small morsels and drops some into his bag.

Oh no. Red flags are going up everywhere, my nutter alarm is flashing on full alert. Why's he doing this? What is going on?

He is mainly pulling out the middle of the sandwiches and dropping them into his bag, but some bread also goes in there. He looks up and sees me staring at him.

"Everything okay?" he asks.

"Yes," I reply.

The background music being played in the restaurant stops for a moment before the next track comes on and I can hear some funny noises. Then the music starts and they disappear beneath the sound of Rod Stewart.

We carry on eating in silence, and he carries on dropping bits of food into his bag, until I can sit in silence no more.

"If you don't mind me asking, why are you putting bits of the food into your bag? If you want to take the food home, we could easily get someone to wrap it up for you. Sorry, it's none of my business, it just seems a bit odd."

"Nothing for you to worry about," he says, as he looks straight at me while pulling the lettuce out of a prawn and salad sandwich and dropping it into his bag. It's as if he thinks that by keeping eye contact, I won't be able to see what's going on.

"You're doing it again," I say. "Is everything OK?"

"Of course," he replies.

Then he sighs unnecessarily loudly and lifts his bag onto the table.

He opens it and inside there are about four guinea pigs, nibbling away on the food he's provided, and squeaking with appreciation.

A look of surprise must cross my face, because he suddenly sounds all aggressive.

"I told you about the pets," he says. "I said I couldn't stay out long because of them."

"Yes, but I thought you meant you had a dog at home or something. I didn't realise they were on the date with us."

"Oh no," he says. "Oh no, look what you've made them do now."

He lifts the bag as urine trickles through it...onto the table...into the little pots of jam and cream laid out before us.

"It's not my fault," I say.

"You frightened them," he counters.

"No, that's not fair," I say. "They were bound to do that. Did it not occur to you that they would do that?"

Ollyver lifts the guinea pigs out of the bag one by one (it turns out there are five of them) and puts them onto the table. "I'm going to clean this bag out, please look after them," he says, disappearing into the men's loos.

Bloody hell.

I glance up and everyone in the café is staring at me; I glance down and the guinea pigs are leaving droppings across the table, nibbling at sandwiches and causing mayhem with the cream. I have no idea what to do. One starts to climb onto the cake stand thing and another has climbed off the table onto one of the shelves next to us on which there are various expensive looking ornaments. Before I can bring the squeaking, little furry thing down, it knocks over a candle and runs to the far side. As I stand up to pick him up and bring him back onto the table, another has joined him and has nestled himself on top of a rather expensive-looking Victorian-style dish. I look back at the table and see the two on the table still nibbling away at the sandwiches on the bottom layer of the stand.

Two?

There were five. Where the hell is the other one? I bring down the two guinea pigs from the shelf before they cause serious damage, and look around for the other one. He's nowhere to be seen. There are now four guinea pigs when there should be five. They're all squeaking and squawking, while a small crowd has gathered.

"I'm sorry, Madam, you can't have pets in the restaurant," says the lovely, floury owner.

"They're not mine, and I seem to have lost one. Can anyone see him anywhere?"

Everyone in the restaurant is now nervously looking around their table legs for a stray pet. But the animal can't be seen anywhere.

"I can see him," says a young boy in a red sweatshirt. "There, look..." He points at my handbag. My lovely, designer handbag. The only nice handbag I own. There's a furry head sticking up - all whiskers and tiny little chirping sounds. I put him back onto the table and zip up my handbag, thanking the boy for his help, then I stand up and pace around the table, marshalling the animals to make sure they don't leave it.

I feel like a farmer trying to control his sheep, except farmers don't have angry diners staring at them, and angry restaurant owners glaring at them while they work.

Ollyver finally returns, and a feeling of relief washes through me.

Now he can take responsibility for them.

"All clean," he says, taking a handful of fresh straw from a side pocket and sprinkling it into the bag. He lifts the guinea pigs one by one and puts them back in, zipping up the top and placing the bag on the floor.

"Where were we?" he says, reaching out for a scone. The table looks like a war zone. The urine that went into the jam has meant the jam running out of its pot and all over the table. The cream has guinea pig droppings in, the table cloth is wet with urine and the sandwiches have been nibbled at by his rodents.

"I'm full, actually," I say, standing up. I hand him the £20 I have tucked inside my phone case for my share of the food and head towards the door.

"Oh, fine," he shouts after me. "Leave if you want to...All the more for me, Andy, Pandy, Mandy, Sandy and Candy."

I glance apologetically at the owner and rush through the door. Joy of greatest joys, there's a bus just coming around the corner which goes vaguely near my house, so I jump onto it and settle into my seat, opening my bag to drop my phone into it. But when I put my hand in, the bag is wet, and the guinea pig has left me a little present: two droppings sit on my makeup bag.

How many dates are there left to go? There can't be too many more, can there?

EIGHTH DATE: RICHARD

"This one could be barefoot," says Juan with a gentle nudge.

"Oh God, why might he be barefoot?" I ask.

"Because of his occupation… He just might be, that's all."

"What is his occupation? You're allowed to tell me that, aren't you? What is he, some sort of Buddhist leader? Or yoga teacher or something?"

"No, actually he is a poet. "

"Oh… That sounds interesting. A poet? I like the sound of that. I wonder whether he'll write a poem about me?"

"He might do. Though I've tried to google his poems and I can't find anything on the internet about him."

"So, he's not a poet, then?"

"Yes, he is, he runs poetry slams, which are where people go and recite their own poetry, at pubs all around the place, mainly in East London… You know, Shoreditch and places like that… Hoxton… All the really trendy places."

"Oh, right. Where am I meeting him?"

"You're meeting him in Richmond Park, at a little café that he says inspired his greatest poem. Do you want me to come and hover in the background?"

"No - honestly, no need at all. I just need to work out what on earth to wear to go to Richmond Park with a poet."

"Wear whatever you want, angel, you're not trying to impress him, you're going to meet him and see whether the two of you get on. Just wear that dress that you wore when you went out with the nutty bloke with the dead wife."

"Oh, you've changed your tune. What happened to 'you have to dress up, or he won't dress up' which will mean he'll arrive with his balls hanging out?"

"I've changed my mind on that now. I realise that there are a lot of fools out there, and whether you wear leggings or smart trousers won't change that. The cream dress looks lovely though."

"Yes, I love that dress, but it hasn't brought me the greatest amount of success so far."

"Well maybe, my dear, this will be your day."

So, I jump on the R68 bus and google 'poetry slams' while the bus winds its way through Twickenham and into Richmond. Juan has given me a picture of Richard the poet, and he looks very normal – like a bank clerk or something. I expected him to look more like Jesus, with flowing hair and an amazing beard, and maybe robes and open-toed sandals or something. Definitely smelling of patchouli oil, and wearing a look of quiet contemplation at all times.

The guy in the photo looks like the sort of guy who would deal with your gas bills, or check how far overdrawn you've gone.

I arrive at the Isabella Café a couple of minutes early, and can see a man sitting on his own. He doesn't look a great deal like the guy in my picture, nor does he look like my fantasy of what a poet should look like, but he is the only guy sitting on his own, so I wander up to him.

"Hi, I'm Mary. Are you Richard?" I say. He jumps and looks at me all alarmed.

"Yes, what do you want?" he says. The man looks absolutely terrified.

"We are supposed to be meeting for a date."

"Are we?"

"Well, if you're Richard, and you're waiting to see someone called Mary, then – yes – we are supposed to be on a date."

"Jolly good," he says. "I'll go and get us some tea, shall I?"

"That would be lovely," I say, as he walks off towards the counter.

He arrives back a few minutes later with a large glass pot full of leaves and petals and two teacups.

"This is rose tea," he says.

It doesn't look very nice. I mean the leaves and petals in the teapot look nice, but the colour of the water is just like urine. It doesn't look as if it will taste very nice and I quite fancy a nice cup of proper tea.

"All the leaves in the tea are from flowers in the park," he says.

"Oh, that's lovely." I like the sound of that. I'll give it a go and see what it tastes like.

"So, I hear you're a poet?" I say.

"Yes. I've always been a poet. Would you like to hear some?"

"Oh, I'd love to," I say, thinking what fun this is going to be.

"I'm a performance poet," he says, jumping to his feet and

coughing loudly. He then proceeds to recite a poem that makes no sense at all but seems to involve him waving his arms around and whooshing like the wind before stomping and howling and shouting and then screaming and falling to the ground shouting, "Do not bury me. Do not bury me, good lord. Do not bury me." The whole café has gone quiet. I look around and see that everyone is staring. The waitress has come over to check he is all right. Richard stays in his position on the floor, lying still, murmuring.

"I'm absolutely fine," he says. "The poem demands that I finish with a murmur."

"Oh," says the waitress. "Well as long as you're all right and don't need an ambulance or anything."

"I'm fine," he says, getting to his feet.

"She ruined that a little bit, didn't she?" he says. "I didn't get to do the full murmur. Shall I do it again?"

"No," I say quickly. "The whole thing was lovely, I got to see it all, don't worry."

"Well, if you're sure," he says. And he sits down opposite me and pours us both a cup of rather nasty weak-looking tea.

"I could show you some more poems," he says. "Perhaps it would be better if you read them instead of me performing them."

"Yes, I think that would be much better," I say.

He brings out a binder full of laminated copies of his poems, and asks me to read and critique them. I'm not convinced I'm going to like any of them, and I have no plans to offer him any sort of critique of them.

"I've only ever asked one date to read my poetry," he says, as I scan through the rather miserable poems about death and the end of the world.

"She said she didn't like them, so I sent her a picture of me cutting myself with blood everywhere, titled, 'I bleed for you.'"

"Oh," I say. "Well, I think these poems are wonderful. All of them. You're very talented."

I haven't read them; I'm just scanning through the self-indulgent dirges and pretending to think they're good in order to avoid any 'cutting'.

"Which is your favourite?" he asks, adding, "I'm so glad you love them."

"It's hard to say. They are all my favourites."

"But if you had to pick one."

"Oh, then the first one," I say, turning back to it. 'The missions of death.'

"Ah, good choice," he says. "Shall we go for a walk through the gardens?"

"Sure," I say. Remarkably, I seem to have gotten away with that.

The two of us head off into the gardens and, to be fair to him, we have a nice time. It's such a beautiful park, full of bushes blooming with flowers of lipstick pink and cherry red, a small brook and gorgeous wildflowers. He shows me his favourite trees and the plants he loves to come and look at every day when he's writing. He buys me an ice-cream and we walk some more.

It's all quite pleasant...walking along with an amiable poet. Then he stops in his tracks and starts shouting at the sky. "Hateful beasts," he howls. "You are all hateful beasts."

"Everything OK?" I ask.

"No, not really. The birds are being very rude to me. Very rude indeed."

"Oh."

"Can you hear them?" he says, before looking up at the sky again.

"I was talking to Mary, not you. Stop interrupting. No, I will not lie down and let you peck me. Just go away."

"Maybe we should go back to the café," I say.

"Yes," he says. "The birds have ruined everything. YET AGAIN."

NINTH DATE: SAM

This whole week has been exhausting – I mean it's just left me feeling so drained and tired, I can hardly think straight.

I don't ever want to tell any strange men about my relationship history or what I'm looking for in a partner ever again.

I've now just got one more date to get through, then – if Juan is right – I will either have met the man of my dreams or I'll be very sure of what I do and don't want from a man. I think he might be right in that I've managed to establish quite clearly what I don't want out of a man. I don't want to go on playdates with five-year olds, I don't want people who are obsessed with their dead wives, keep piles of papers in their flats or run away when they see me. Oh, and a man who hasn't had his gloved hand inside me; that would be nice. That can't be too much to ask, surely?

Maybe today's date will provide a man who becomes my life

partner. Well, it's worth trying. The guy I am meeting is called Sam; he describes himself as "big and cuddly", and wants to meet a woman who is like him. I think that description fits me like a glove, so hopefully we're going to get on. We are meeting at a bar in the middle of Kingston, which I'm not keen on, but we're going to the cinema.

I push my way into the Kings Tonne pub and through the throngs of young people (by "young" I really mean "under age"). When I get to the bar, I see a gorgeous big man with a lovely, wide smiling face looking at me.

"Wow! You must be Mary," he says. And for the first time in this whole internet dating experience I feel a real rush of attraction. A lot of the guys I've met have been nice, but I haven't really fancied any of them. This guy though - he's really nice. He reminds me a little bit of Ted, but I try to push that to the back of my mind. He's got a lovely open face, big shiny eyes and looks genuinely thrilled to see me.

"And you must be Sam," I say, smiling back at him as he grabs me in a big bear hug.

"What can I get you to drink then, gorgeous?" he says, and I feel like all these ridiculous dates have been worth it – here is a genuinely lovely guy.

He picks up our drinks. "After you," he says, as we head over to a table that he has reserved by throwing his jacket and jumper across it.

We sit down with our drinks. "Sorry to make you lead the way, but I wanted to sneakily look at you as you walked. I didn't expect you to be so gorgeous," he says. "I love the way you are dressed."

He looks me up and down as he talks and I feel myself blush under his intense gaze.

"You look lovely, too," I say, slightly embarrassed now.

He is still appraising me, as his eyes alight on my shoes. I've got cream open toe sandals on, not very high – just kitten heels, but he clearly likes them a lot.

"You have such beautiful feet. I love your shoes," he says.

"Thank you." I'm not sure what else to say.

"And that colour on your toenails," he adds. Then he looks at my face and can see that I'm feeling quite awkward.

"Sorry," he says. "You just look great. But I've already said that, haven't I? I'll stop saying it now."

We finish our drinks while chatting about all manner of things… what's happening in the news, friends we have, and places we both know. We do that thing of talking about places we know and trying to work out whether we've both been there at the same time. Then we decide to have another drink even though it's almost time for the cinema. "We'll have to drink this one really fast," he says, standing up and heading for the bar.

"I'll get these," I say.

"No, you won't. You stay there. I'll be back in a minute."

He heads to the bar while I sit there and watch him, smiling to myself at how nice he is. I'm dying to tell Juan and Dave how complimentary he's being. The two them have said a few times that they think men would get on much better with women if they just gave them compliments every so often.

"Here we go," he says, putting my drink down on the table. He has enormous, hairy hands and is quite tanned. He looks almost Mediterranean with his glossy black hair, but says he was born in Manchester, and his parents moved down south when he was young.

"Why don't you swing round," he says, pulling my chair so

that I'm facing him next to me. I'm very impressed that he can swing me round like that. I notice his eyes have moved down my legs, and he's staring at my feet again. He really loves my shoes. It's bizarre.

"I'll try and get some in your size if you want," I say, and he bursts out laughing.

"I don't think the shoes would look half as nice with my big hairy ugly feet in them. I do really like your feet though...they are all soft and fleshy and lovely."

Fleshy? Really? Is that a good word? Is he saying I have fat feet?

"Come on then, we have to neck these," he says. "The film starts in ten minutes and we are five minutes from the cinema. Are you ready?"

"I'm ready," I say, and we both down our drinks straight away.

I've only got a small glass of wine but he's got a pint of beer, so he has the biggest struggle, but he seems to do it OK... knocking the drink back and standing up with an appreciative grunt. "Come on then, let's go."

At the cinema, I step in front of him and head to the counter.

"I'm buying the tickets," I say. "You bought all the drinks."

"Too late," he declares. "I bought them this morning. Here you go..."

He holds out tickets, not just for the normal cinema seats, but for the posh seats in the row with the lovely velvety backs that cost extra.

"Oh, you're spoiling me," I say, and he gives me a gentle squeeze as we walk towards screen two.

The auditorium is quite busy, but as usual there are no

people sitting in the posh seats, so we walk up to them and take our places, sitting in splendid isolation on our velvet thrones.

"This is nice," he says. "We've got the row to ourselves. I hope I can trust you to keep your hands off me."

"Ha ha ha," I say, tucking my handbag under my seat, and stretching my legs out in front. "It's lovely. Having all this room is great," I say.

"Yes, I love it when you stretch your legs out like that."

"You're not going to start going on about my shoes again, are you?"

"It's not your shoes that entice me, it's your feet. I love women's feet, and yours are amazing."

"Oh, right," I say. What else can you say? I mean what on earth do you say to a man who says that?

"Would you mind if I removed your shoes?" he whispers, as the lights go down and the screen flickers into life, asking people to turn off their mobile phones.

"I think I'll just leave them on," I say.

"Please," he says. "I did buy all the drinks and the cinema ticket, the least you could do is let me touch your feet."

"You're making me feel really awkward," I say. "Can we watch the film and stop talking about my feet?"

"But they're so beautiful. I just love larger ladies with painted toenails. It drives me wild."

While the adverts dance across the screen, telling us of films that are coming soon, I sit there, nervously, with my feet tucked under, while Sam sits there peering down at the bits of my feet he can see.

"It should be against the law to hide feet as gorgeous as that," he says. "Beautiful, sexy feet should be seen, not tucked away."

I decide to ignore him, and just concentrate on the film, but

I have to tell you that it's very hard to ignore a man who insists on going on, and on, and on about your feet.

The film starts and we fall into a companionable silence. Thank God. He's stopped the bloody fat lady foot fetish for a moment.

But...not for long. Just as I've forgotten about his madness, and am starting to enjoy the film, he starts shuffling about and drops his keys on the floor.

"Excuse me," he says, clambering down and fishing around for them. "They're here somewhere."

Then I feel my toes getting wet. What's happening? I look down and he's sucking my toes through my shoes. Sucking my toes! Have you ever had that happen to you while you're in the cinema? No, you haven't. And you know why? Because you haven't been internet dating with a mad chubby chaser. And neither will I. EVER AGAIN. I kick out to push him off and end up booting him rather sharply in the face.

"Ahhh..." he cries, standing up. "What is wrong with you?"

"What is wrong with *me*?" I ask. "The question is - what is wrong with *you*? What nutter starts sucking a woman's toes through her shoes, in the cinema?"

"It's what I like doing," he says, sounding pitiful now. We're standing there in the middle of the cinema, in the posh row. No-one has told us to be quiet but I suspect that's because they are enjoying the performance. It's not every day you see a man sucking a fat lady's shoes in the cinema and her kicking him in the face.

We leave the auditorium and go to the lobby. As soon as we are in the light, I can see that he has blood running all the way down his face.

"You should go to hospital," I say. "I'm going home."

And I turn and walk out of the door.

NINE DATES IN TWO WEEKS, BUT WHAT HAVE WE LEARNED?

I am sitting, glass of wine in hand, back in my flat, tucked up in the armchair while Dave, Juan and Charlie sit opposite on the sofa, open-mouthed as I recall the events of the evening.

Dave looks at Juan, then at Charlie. "What sort of characteristics were you looking for in the ideal man when you set up these dates?" he asks. "I mean – every one of them was operating at a whole new level of bonkers."

"I know," says Juan, scratching his head. "They all seemed like nice guys on paper."

"The police should sign you up when they are looking for people who have committed particularly insane crimes – you'd find them in a heartbeat. You have a madman detector of some sort."

"Yeah," he says again. "I don't know what to say. I feel awful."

"Hey, don't worry – it was fine," I say. "It was a huge learning experience."

"Yep – you learned never to let Juan pick out dates for you again." Dave says.

"No – come on – it's not Juan's fault. There are a lot of nutters out there."

"Yes, but – honestly – to get that many lunatics – one after the other…date after date. That's odd."

"It's unfair to say they were all lunatics. The first guy was completely nice, it was just that he hadn't gotten over his wife."

"I'm sure there are a lot of guys out there who lose their wives and struggle to get over it – but they don't take future dates on a pilgrimage to see where she died."

"But I don't think he meant it like that: he didn't mean it in a threatening or angry way; we'd just been talking about it and we happened to be passing it, so he pointed it out."

"No, Mary, that's not true…he turned completely the wrong way at the roundabout in order to take you there, and you had to ask him to take you home. Dead Wife Darren is a nutter – plain and simple. Don't you agree, Juan?"

"It's very hard to disagree when you put it like that," he says, sheepishly.

"Which guy came next?" asks Dave.

"The guy who ran away," I say.

"Well – he was just rude," says Juan. "A horrible, rude man."

"Yes – he was rude rather than mad," says Dave. "But I did enjoy the descriptions of him legging it like Usain Bolt while Juan screamed obscenities after him in Spanish. Well done, Juan. I wish I'd been there to support you."

The two men high five one another, and ask me which date came after that.

"Oh – that was Martin who took me on a playdate. Remember him?"

"I remember all the little boys crying when you left because they enjoyed playing Action Man games with you. And – yes, he was mad, but it was Harry the hoarder after that – and he was all your doing," Juan says to me. "That one was nothing to do with me."

"I accept full responsibility for that particular nutter," I say. "I still can't get over what his flat was like – there must have been about thirty piles of newspapers, some of the ones in the corridor went up to the ceiling. And the cutlery...I've never known anyone get so excited about cutlery. It was weird on a whole new scale. But he seemed so nice and normal until we went back to his place. That was very odd, and very disappointing."

I get up and top everyone's glasses up, while Charlie tries to work out who was next. "Oh, it was Ollyver with his guinea pigs," she says, looking up from the print outs in front of her. "There was no sign of him being a nutter on his profile. It mentions pets in the 'things I like' section, but it doesn't say that he'll be taking his guinea pigs with him or anything. He doesn't even mention his pets in the main piece he's written about himself, it just appears at the end. It's bizarre."

"That was the only date on which I felt really uncomfortable," I say. "On most of them I got out of there quickly, before it became a mad disaster, but when those guinea pigs were all over the table and he went to the loo to wash his bag out, I swear to God, I don't think I've ever felt so much pressure in my life before – they were running everywhere, causing chaos. And he just wanted to carry on afterwards like nothing had happened, even though there were guinea pig droppings all over the bloody food."

"Richard the poet was after that, then the mad chubby chaser." Charlie says.

"Richard was fine," I say. "He just loved to perform poetry. I didn't fancy him at all, and he didn't fancy me, but when we went for a walk it was really nice because he knew all the names of the trees and flowers, and had lots of stories about historical encounters in the park. I enjoyed that date, once he'd stopped going on about his poems, and until he started screaming that the birds were being rude to him."

"And the madman at the end?"

"Yep, tonight was odd. I kicked him really hard, you know. I didn't mean to, but he took me by such surprise, I lashed out. I wouldn't be surprised if I broke his nose."

"Serves him right," says Dave. "Bloody idiot."

Charlie and Juan have been unusually quiet during this conversation, except to defend themselves from time to time.

"It was all fun, though. Thanks for trying. Here's to great friends who try to help you meet someone..."

I raise my glass and Dave raises his, adding: "Even if the men they fix you up with are stark, staring mad." Then Juan and Charlie glance at one another and tentatively raise their glasses.

"I think I may have cocked up a bit," says Juan, lowering his head.

"No, don't be silly, I'm fine," I say. "It was good fun, we're only joking."

"No, not about the dates per se," he says. "I mean about something else that I have planned."

There's a sort of silence, because if he's not embarrassed about the dates, but he is embarrassed about something else he's planned then this something else must be quite special.

"What have you done?" I say, looking at both of them.

"Well we've kind of organised something for Saturday night."

"What have you organised for Saturday night?"

"A party."

"Oh, that's nice."

"Yes," says Charlie. "Only I now think it's maybe not very nice. In fact, it may be the most stupid idea ever. We thought of having a little get together because of Juan leaving and everything, but then we got a bit carried away…"

"What have you done?" I ask.

"Well, we've sort of invited all the people you dated to it."

"You what?"

"Sorry. We just didn't think they'd all be as mad as they have been. At the beginning, we sent them invitations to a party at Charlie's house on Saturday."

Dave looks like he'll explode with surprise and sheer incomprehension, Charlie looks sheepish and Juan is looking around the room, refusing to meet anyone's eye.

A party at which all the nutters that I have dated over the past week will be together…hoarder, sprinter, toe sucker and poet. And will there be guinea pigs and a five-year-old child there?

Bloody hell, this is insane.

"There's something else we need to tell you," says Charlie.

"What?"

"Ted is seeing someone."

"Ted? What, my Ted?"

"Yes, I'm really sorry, angel. I bumped into Veronica who said she saw him with Michella from Fat Club in the pub near him. I don't know whether it's serious or anything, but I thought I should tell you."

Charlie keeps talking, but I don't hear anything else. I feel like I've been shot. It's like I'm falling through the gaps in the universe. My head is spinning and I can't get enough air into my lungs. Has someone turned off the oxygen?

Suddenly, the party feels neither here nor there. I don't care whether there's a party or not. I couldn't give a flying fuck whether those losers are congregating or not. I just want Ted.

"But I love him," I say, standing up and heading to my bedroom before the tears come. "I love him like I've never loved anyone before."

THE PARTY TO END ALL PARTIES

It's a difficult couple of days after hearing about Ted. I feel I'm existing in a different reality to everyone else… operating on the torn edges of life…all meandering and vague. I awake in the early hours of the morning, and am desperate to sleep in the afternoons: it's as if I've just been on a long-distance flight. I don't know what to do with myself. My mind whirs so much that it hurts and images of Ted and the great times we had together flash aggressively into my mind suddenly and without warning. I find myself relying on the kindness of Juan and Charlie during these difficult early days, as they spend hours talking to me and making sure I'm able to function.

I tell them to go ahead with the party, because I can't face telling them to cancel it. It feels easier to go ahead with everything and somehow cope with it, than it does to make a drama about stopping it.

So, the day arrives, and I am determined to put my broken

heart to one side, and try to enjoy myself: this is Juan's going away party, and there's every chance that none of the daters will turn up. It could be just a few of us, drinking wine and celebrating our friendship.

On the other hand, if they do turn up, it will be the most ridiculous party ever to be thrown.

Juan is still reeling with amazement that I allowed the party to take place. In a bizarre way, if it hadn't been for discovering that Ted was dating Michella, I probably wouldn't have. But that news wounded me so badly and destabilised me to such an extent that I feel nothing can hurt me now.

"Are you OK?" Juan asks me for the one-thousandth time and I tell him I'm fine, but I still think it will be a ridiculous party.

"It depends what you mean by "ridiculous party". I think the most ridiculous parties are the best parties."

"Well, this one should be a belter then," I say.

At 7pm, we head to Charlie's place. We are all glammed up and ready to party. Juan is in a sparkly striped suit that is extremely tight. He looks magnificent, of course, even if his hair is all standing on end making him look as if he's been lifted out of a well by his ankles.

"You need more lipstick," he says. "I'm going to be your beauty consultant for the evening."

I notice that Juan is wearing makeup himself. He is wearing eyeliner which he insists on calling "guy liner", and definitely has foundation on even though he denies it. He produces a gorgeous cherry red lipstick that Charlie has handed to him and proceeds to apply it. I'm sure I look like a bloody clown, but there's too much else to worry about with the prospect of the attendees at the party tonight, so I just let him put it on me.

Charlie looks gorgeous. I mean – really lovely. She's wearing a cream sheath dress and has bare legs which are all fake tanned and glossy. They look so long and elegant with her high, gold, strappy sandals. If I wore them for more than five minutes, I'd be flat on my face - I'm not good with high heels - but I'm confident that Charlie will be striding around the party looking like a supermodel.

I'm already starting to reconsider offering to take her on my free trip to Saint Lucia. I can't imagine how gorgeous she is going to look in a bikini, and how correspondingly awful I will look.

"You look like Marilyn Monroe with that lipstick on," she says. I smile at her, and don't offer the retort that Marilyn Monroe has been dead for about fifty years. Instead I thank her, and we walk sheepishly out of the flat.

"It's very nice of you to host this," I say to Charlie, and she drapes her arm over my shoulder as we walk down the path to her flat.

"You're very welcome."

"Do you think any of the mad daters will turn up?"

"I think some will," she replies.

"What about Usain Bolt?"

"Who?"

"You know, the guy who ran away at the speed of light as soon as he saw me."

"Oh blimey, Usain. Yes. I don't know. I wouldn't have thought so after the abuse we gave him."

"You know this party is the most ridiculous idea ever, don't you?"

"Yes," says Charlie. "When we thought of it, we imagined you going on lots of light, friendly dates and not being sure who you liked best, so we thought that if we invited them all to a party, you'd be able to decide. We never once imagined that there would be so many nutters."

"Maybe we could have a sign, so that if I'm talking to someone who is driving me bonkers, I can signal to you, somehow?"

"Good plan," says Juan, appearing at my side. "Maybe just bash your hands on your head and squeal or something?"

"I think it might call for something more subtle than that," I say. "I have this amazing Great Aunt Millicent. She hates meetings and parties, so we have this thing where, if she is stuck with someone who is boring her, she just wiggles her ear lobe, and I look out for it and when I spot it, I go on over and save her."

"Let's do that," Charlie says. "That's a good plan"

"She is just the loveliest, most astonishingly interesting person ever. I don't see her very often because she moved to New York, but mum says she's moving back over here, and I can't wait to catch up with her. She is about ninety now, but still dresses as if she's going to the state opening of Parliament or a royal wedding or something, you know – always immaculate."

There is a loud banging on the door just as I'm about to go storming into a few of Millicent's incredible stories. My heart beats a little faster, and I push past Charlie into the kitchen and pour myself the largest glass of wine imaginable.

"Don't worry, it's only Dave," shouts Juan. "You can put the cyanide down."

"Oh darling," come Juan's unmissable tones. He pops his head into the kitchen. "This is going to be the best party ever. I mean...it's brilliant... Don't you think?"

"Brilliant? Let's just see how it goes, shall we?" I say.

It's a bizarre thing, but part of me is really embracing the madness of all this as a huge distraction from the pain of Ted having found someone new. I felt strangled by the knowledge that he has a girlfriend a couple of days ago, but the riotous ludicrousness of this party is filling my mind and stopping the darker thoughts from entering it. I'm sort of grateful that it's going on, even though I'm actually dreading the reality of seeing these bizarre men again.

The first date to arrive at the party is Martin. Dave looks at me quizzically and I mouth, "play date". He puts his thumbs up in recognition of the fact that he now realises that this is the guy who took me on a date to a toddler's café party, and left me playing games with the children while he chatted to the mums, until Charlie and Juan turned up to rescue me.

"Lovely to see you again," he says, kissing me gently on either cheek and shaking hands with the others when I introduce them.

"I remember you from the café," he says to Juan. "Why did you have to leave so suddenly, Mary?"

"Well, it was a bit odd," I say. "You know – going to play with children when we were supposed to be on a date."

"Yes, but I had a son. I said in my profile that I had a son. He's part of the package. I didn't want to leave him at home. Sorry – but I thought it would work as a simple, relaxed first date."

"Yes, but – it was hard for us to talk properly."

"I know. I suppose I was thinking that those serious face-to-face dinners when you first know someone can be so intense. I thought we might have fun if we bonded over Lego or something. I thought that if we got on in a relaxed environment like that, we could then go out more formally later. But you just rushed off."

"Yes, because it all seemed so odd."

"I'm really sorry you found it odd. It's completely my fault, I misjudged everything. Still, it's lovely to be invited here to meet up with you again."

"Yes, you too," I say.

Well, maybe that one wasn't a nutter after all.

As I'm standing there, enjoying this man's company in a way that I never expected to, it dawns on me that I don't know whether he knows that I went on lots of internet dates, and they have all been invited tonight.

"Have you two me?" I say, introducing him to Dave, and asking Dave whether he would get him a drink.

I walk over to Juan, and take him aside. "Do these men know that there will be lots of men at this party who I have dated?"

"Of course not," replies Juan. "Why would I tell them that?"

"Because when they find out they might be cross?"

"Well, tough, they haven't been exactly the most glorious of men. This party is for you, not them."

As Juan and I talk, I see Ollyver arrive. He has a bag with him, which immediately makes me panic. The last thing we need here are guinea pigs running all over the flat. Behind him comes Harry, the guy who had seemed so lovely when I met him in the bar, but then thoroughly weird in his flat – with his piles of newspapers, boxes and boxes of rubbish, and general weirdness about cutlery. He comes in and stands with his hands on his hips, surveying the scene. Then he sees me and walks over.

"Thanks for inviting me," he says. "I was very surprised to be invited to a party. I thought I might have blown it with the text I sent."

"Of course not, we can be friends," I say. But inside I'm thinking, blew it with the text? Mate, you blew it well before the text.

I introduce him to Juan and the two men shake hands, before he wanders into the kitchen to get a drink. Juan turns to me.

"He seems really nice," he says. "Which one was he? Why didn't you like him?"

"He is the one I met in the pub, remember, the one who is a hoarder."

"Oh yes, I remember now," says Juan. "It's a shame – nice guy. Good firm handshake. He's obviously quite strong."

"Yes, from lifting all those damn newspapers."

I walk into the kitchen to get a refill and stumble across the oddest of scenes.

Martin is holding Ollyver's guinea pig while Ollyver fills up Harry's glass. Of course, it's only a matter of time until one of them says "so, how do you know Mary?" And the whole thing will implode, and they will realise what this party is all about. I look over at Dave and give him a warm smile. I think I might need him to get me safely out of here if things kick off.

Next into the fray is Dead Wife Darren, arriving just before Rupert, my gynaecologist (there's a sentence I never imagined saying). Now it's getting weird. If anyone asks him how he knows me, I'm not sure whether he'll say, "I'm her gynaecologist," or "I met her on a blind date." Either one is ridiculous, but I think the former is more ridiculous, so I hope he says that we went on a date.

I look over at Charlie and realise she's talking to someone

that I vaguely know. It's one of the date men, but I can't quite work out which one it is, especially since he has bandages across his face. It looks like he's been in a nasty accident.

"Well, this is very nice. Thank you very much for inviting me," says Rupert, forcing me to spin round. I smile at him and we exchange kisses on the cheek. "I thought I'd never see you again," he says.

"Well, not until my next smear test, eh?"

"It's unlikely to be me that does it," he says. "You know, you really shouldn't worry quite so much about my occupation. I'm a nice guy. We seem to get on well. I didn't quite understand why you ran away."

"You didn't understand?"

"Well, I did, I just didn't think there was any need for it. I think we could've had another drink and carried on chatting."

"I just felt so embarrassed," I said. It is at that point that I realise who it is that Charlie is talking to. The chubby chaser. The rather rampant and unashamedly foot-obsessed lunatic, and now I remember why he is all bandaged up. I kicked him very hard in the face.

I look over at him and Charlie, and see him looking down at her lovely feet, all on show in her gold open-toe sandals. Oh God. Charlie is very slender, so wouldn't appeal to his chubby chasing but might appeal to him on the foot front. You can practically see all of her feet.

What on earth was she thinking?

"I'm just going to pop over and check Charlie is okay," I say to Rupert. "It's lovely to see you again."

I walk over to Charlie and say hello to Sam. "How is your nose?" I say to him. "I'm sorry I kicked you in the face. It was entirely an accident."

There is a small gasp from Charlie as she realises who this is, and she disappears.

I turn back to Sam. "Seriously, how is your face?"

"Feeling much better now, thank you very much," he says. "I'm sorry about the way I behaved. It was unforgivable. The main reason I came today was to apologise and tell you that I was completely out of order."

But, as we're talking, I notice his gaze stray to the other side of the room. I follow the direction of his eyes and see that the ladies from Fat Club have arrived. This must be absolute paradise to our resident chubby chaser.

"They are my friends," I say. "Just try and be normal and friendly, please."

"Of course, I will," he says. "I have already explained that my behaviour before was an aberration. Totally out of character." But then he pushes past me and makes a beeline for the chubbiest ladies at the party.

I'm standing there alone, when Rupert appears again. "Is it actually your birthday today?" he says.

"No - the party is because Juan is going back to Spain soon, so we thought we'd get a few people together."

"Oh, I see," he says. "I assumed that Juan was your brother, is that not the case?"

I look over at Juan, who weighs less than my arm, and has a distinctively Mediterranean look. I'm a very fat English lady with rosy cheeks and highlighted blonde hair. It's hard to imagine two people looking less similar. I've no idea how anyone on earth could think that we were brother and sister.

"He's a friend I met on holiday," I say. "A really lovely guy. We stayed in touch."

I start to stroke my ear, worried that Rupert will think I'm interested if I hang around him too long. He's a nice guy, but I swear to God I can't possibly date my gynaecologist. It's too weird. And...the undeniable truth is - I don't fancy him in the least.

My ear rubbing brings Charlie quickly to my side, but then the two of us hear a small commotion, and the sound of Dave's raised voice. "What the fuck?" he shouts, before there is a scream from Veronica, one of my friends from Fat Club, and the sound of people scampering out of the kitchen.

"She's got rats," says Veronica, tossing her glossy dark hair over her shoulders and fleeing the room. "Your friend has rats."

"I bloody haven't," says Charlie, who has never taken much to Veronica. She storms into the kitchen to see what's going on. "It's that mad bastard with his guinea pigs," she says. "They are running all around the kitchen. Oh God."

I head into the kitchen to help Charlie and stumble upon a scene that I never expected to witness. Harry the hoarder and Martin Playdate are on their hands and knees crawling around with Ollyver trying to catch his squeaking pets.

"There, over by you," shouts Harry. "In that corner, right next to your knee. Have you got it?"

"Yes, got it," says Martin, standing up and holding the fluffy little animal aloft, like it's the World Cup or something.

"Ah, it's Candy," says Ollyver, taking her and putting her straight into his bag. "I think Candy is my favourite. She understands me in a way that the others don't. But then she's older than they are."

"Right," says Harry. "Well I'm glad she's safely back with you, then."

"How many are there?" I say, noticing that the men have got

back onto their hands and knees and are still searching. "And why do you have to take them wherever you go?"

"Because I don't like to leave them at home all day on their own," he replies aggressively. "Two escaped; one has just been returned to the fold, meaning one is still missing."

"Got it," says Martin, seizing hold of the other runaway pet. "I'm good at this, aren't I? Really good at it."

"Yes, very good," I reply. Perhaps he should put 'guinea pig catcher' on his CV?

"Oh hello, what have we got here?" says Richard the poet, striding in and observing the scene. "I didn't realise it was a 'bring a rat' party."

"It's not a rat," shout Ollyver and Charlie at the same time, with Charlie adding, "I don't have rats in my house, OK?"

"OK," says Richard. "No rats... good for you. I have a poem about small animals, actually. Let me recite it for you."

Now, as we know, Richard can't just recite a poem, so as soon as he says this, I know there's going to be an over-the-top performance coming up. But I don't anticipate anything like what follows.

Richard jumps up, so he is standing on top of the table under which the guinea pig hunters have been conducting their search.

"Be careful; you might fall," I caution.

"No, I won't. This table and I are friends. Anyway, I regard gravity as an impertinent con trick unworthy of being taken seriously."

And, with that, he begins his dramatic tale.

"Mini monsters, scary faces, long of hair, in creepy places."

Then he pauses, jumps up and down, landing noisily on the table top, and shouts at the top of his voice: "Oh, you evil, feckless, meaningless others. All to damnation – creatures and mothers."

He's howling now, really howling, and most of the party are in the kitchen, trying to work out what's going on.

Charlie and I are madly twirling our earlobes.

"Enough," shouts Dave. "We'd like you to leave."

It's fair to say that we're all done with this now. Done with online dating, done with bonkers parties. Done with it all.

"Do you want me to leave?" asks Richard, confusion written across his face.

"YES," we chorus. "All of you!"

LIFE WITHOUT TED

Once they have gone, I flop onto Charlie's sofa, and sit there in silence.

"Do you think we were too hasty there?" says Juan. "You know – chucking them out like that."

"No," Charlie and Dave say in unison. "We had to get them out. That poet is from another planet."

"Yeah, he's OK when he's not reciting his poems," I say, offering a weak defence of him. "When we went walking in Richmond Park, he was lovely, but those poems he writes...and his need to perform them...Jesus – that's hard-core."

"With hindsight, the party wasn't a great idea, was it?" says Juan.

"Even without hindsight," I say. And that's when we all start laughing.

"How are you feeling, Mary?"

"I'm OK," I say. "I just feel exhausted. And sad, of course. I'm sad I cocked things up so badly with Ted."

"You're assuming you cocked things up. You don't know that. Why don't you just call him and see how he feels."

"Yes," I say, but it's breaking me in two that he might be with Michella, or someone like that. Mich is a woman we met at Fat Club...she's a younger, slimmer, prettier version of me. I became convinced he was seeing her. I was wrong, but perhaps things have changed? I don't want to call him and be brutally rejected by him. My efforts to contact him before backfired magnificently.

"I need to work out how to get Ted back," I say, in barely more than a whisper.

"I know," says Charlie. "We'll all work out how to get him back." She cuddles me then, and Juan joins in...the three of us all wrapped round each other after the silliest party ever. Dave looks on, and then piles in with us.

"You will get him back," says Juan. "I can feel it in my bones."

Will Mary be reunited with Ted? Read the next books in the series to find out. In *Adorable Fat Girl and the Six-Week Transformation,* and *The Reunion,* we find out once and for all whether Mary and Ted will end up together...

FANCY READING THE NEXT INSTALMENT?

ADORABLE FAT GIRL AND THE SIX-WEEK TRANSFORMATION

UK: My Book

US: My Book

Can Mary Brown lose weight, smarten up and look fabulous enough to win back the love of her life? And can she do it in just six weeks?

In this romantic comedy from the award-winning, best-selling, Adorable Fat Girl series, our luscious heroine goes all out to try and win back the affections of Ted, her lovely ex-boyfriend. She becomes convinced that the way to do it is by putting herself through a six-week transformation plan in time for her friend's 30th birthday party that Ted is coming to. But, like most things in Mary Brown's life, things don't go exactly according to plan.

Featuring drunk winter Olympics, an amorous fitness

instructor, a crazy psychic, spying, dieting, exercising and a trip to hospital with a Polish man called Lech.

ADORABLE FAT GIRL AND THE REUNION

UK: My Book

US: My Book

You join us at an exciting time...our gorgeous, generously proportioned heroine is about to be reunited with Ted - her lovely, kind, thoughtful, wonderful ex-boyfriend. She is still madly in love with him, but how does he feel about her? Will love blossom once more? Or has Ted moved on and met someone else?

Featuring river boats, a wild psychic, sequined leotards, lots of gossip, fun, silliness and a huge, glorious love story...but is the love story about Ted & Mary or someone else entirely?

ALSO BY BERNICE BLOOM

Books, book & more books

I've written lots of books and there are more coming out all the time!

They are listed below. To find them all, see the Bernice Bloom page on Amazon:

UK: https://www.amazon.co.uk/Bernice-Bloom/e/B01MPZ5SBA/ref=dp_byline_cont_pop_ebooks_1

US: https://www.amazon.com/Bernice-Bloom/e/B01MPZ5SBA/ref=dp_byline_cont_pop_ebooks_1

THE ADORABLE FAT GIRL BOOKS

BOOK ONE: Diary of an Adorable Fat Girl

BOOK TWO: Adventures of an Adorable Fat Girl

BOOK THREE: Crazy Life of an Adorable Fat Girl

BOOK FOUR: Christmas with Adorable Fat Girl

BOOK FIVE: Adorable Fat Girl on Safari

BOOK SIX: Cruise with an Adorable Fat Girl

BOOK SEVEN: Adorable Fat Girl Takes up Yoga

BOOK EIGHT Adorable Fat Girl goes to weight loss camp

BOOK NINE: Adorable Fat Girl goes online dating

BOOK TEN: Adorable Fat Girl and the six-week transformation

BOOK ELEVEN: Adorable Fat Girl in lockdown

BOOK TWELVE: Adorable Fat Girl and the reunion

BOOK THIRTEEN: It's Christmas Again (out in December)

Mary Brown Mysteries

BOOK ONE: Marvellous Mary Brown and the Mysterious Invitation

BOOK TWO: Marvellous Mary Brown & the Manhunt (out in December 2020)

The box sets

BOX SET ONE: First three books combined

BOX SET TWO First three holiday books combined

BOX SET THREE: The first two weight loss books

BOX SET FOUR: Romance books combined (6-week and reunion)

BOX SET FIVE: Mystery books combined (available in December)

BOX SET SIX: Christmas books combined (available in December)

Non-fiction

Adorable Fat Girl shares her Weight Loss Tips

Handbook for Adorable Fat Girls

Look out for the stand alone books:

I'm dating a Hollywood Star!

Mother & Son (out in 2021)

Then there's the **Sunshine Cottage** series about the wonderful Lopez family based in Cove Bay. The first book is out now, and the whole series will be available in 2021

You can find them all by going to the Bernice Bloom page on Amazon:

UK: https://www.amazon.co.uk/Bernice-Bloom/e/B01MPZ5SBA/ref=dp_byline_cont_pop_ebooks_1

US: https://www.amazon.com/Bernice-Bloom/e/B01MPZ5SBA/ref=dp_byline_cont_pop_ebooks_1

Thank you for your incredible support xx

Printed in Great Britain
by Amazon

84379237R10079